Lecture Notes of the Institute for Computer Sciences, Social Informatics and Telecommunications Engineering 253

More information about this series at http://www.springer.com/series/8197

Pietro Cipresso · Silvia Serino
Yuri Ostrovsky · Justin T. Baker (Eds.)

Pervasive Computing Paradigms for Mental Health

7th International Conference, MindCare 2018
Boston, MA, USA, January 9–10, 2018
Proceedings

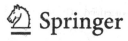 Springer

Editors
Pietro Cipresso
Istituto Auxologico Italiano
Milan
Italy

Silvia Serino
Università Cattolica del Sacro Cuore
Milan
Italy

Yuri Ostrovsky
Massachusetts Institute of Technology
Cambridge, MA
USA

Justin T. Baker
McLean Institute for Technology in
   Psychiatry and Harvard Medical School
Belmont, MA
USA

ISSN 1867-8211   ISSN 1867-822X (electronic)
Lecture Notes of the Institute for Computer Sciences, Social Informatics
and Telecommunications Engineering
ISBN 978-3-030-01092-8   ISBN 978-3-030-01093-5 (eBook)
https://doi.org/10.1007/978-3-030-01093-5

Library of Congress Control Number: 2018934325

This Springer imprint is published by the registered company Springer Nature Switzerland AG
The registered company address is: Gewerbestrasse 11, 6330 Cham, Switzerland

Preface

The incredible diffusion of technology in psychology and neuroscience research and practice has created relevant opportunities, but has also opened new research questions that deserve attention.

This strong synergy between mental health care and technology has found in the Mindcare Symposium a place to meet. In its seven editions, the MindCare Symposium has gathered researchers and practitioners from technological, medical, and psychological disciplines from more than 30 countries creating a strong community to share a common passion for building new computing paradigms and for addressing a multitude of challenges in mental health care.

The 7 International Symposium on Pervasive Computing Paradigms for Mental Health was held at the Massachusetts Institute of Technology's Samberg Conference Center in Cambridge, Massachusetts, in January 2018.

The symposium explored how advanced computing and communication technologies (from the use of wearables sensors and ecological virtual environments, to the use of big data and machine learning techniques or voice-user interfaces) can be used to support and promote well-being through objective continuous data collection and personalized treatments.

Two distinguished keynote speakers, Prof. Giuseppe Riva and Prof. Justin T. Baker, support these reflections with two interesting theoretical proposals investigating the use of technologies in monitoring and maintaining mental health.

We would like to strongly thank Prof. Emilio Bizzi, Emeritus Institute Professor at MIT, for his active participation and discussion during the symposium. We also acknowledge the European-funded project "BodyPass" – API-ecosystem for cross-sectorial exchange of 3D personal data (H2020-779780) — for supporting the event.

Pietro Cipresso
Silvia Serino
Yuri Ostrovsky
Justin T. Baker

Organization

Steering Committee

Steering Committee Chair

Imrich Chlamtac   University of Trento, Italy

Organizing Committee

Local Chairs

Yuri Ostrovsky   Massachusetts Institute of Technology, MA, USA
Justin T. Baker   McLean Institute for Technology in Psychiatry
                      and Harvard Medical School, MA, USA

Symposium General Chairs

Silvia Serino   Catholic University of Milan, Italy
Pietro Cipresso   Istituto Auxologico Itaiiano, Italy

Program Chair

Daniela Villani   Catholic University of Milan, Italy

Publicity Chair

Stefano Triberti   Catholic University of Milan, Italy

Poster Chair

Elisa Pedroli   Istituto Auxologico Italiano, Italy

Web Chair

Desirée Colombo   Universidad de Valencia, Spain

Sponsorship and Exhibits Chair

Elisa Pedroli   Istituto Auxologico Italiano, Italy

Publications Chair

Javier Fernàndez Kirszman   Universidad de Valencia, Spain

Conference Manager

Daniel Miske   EAI - European Alliance for Innovation

Technical Program Committee

Afsaneh Doryab	Carnegie Mellon University, USA
Anja Thieme	Microsoft Research Cambridge, USA
Anouk Keizer	Utrecht University, The Netherlands
Conor Linehan	University of Cork, Ireland
Erik Grönvall	IT University of Copenhagen, Denmark
Francesca Morganti	University of Bergamo, Italy
Francisco Nunes	Universidade Nova de Lisboa, Portugal
Javier Hernandez	MIT Media Lab, USA
Jean Marcel Dos Reis Costa	Cornell University, USA
José Gutiérrez-Maldonado	Universidad de Barcelona, Spain
Julian Childs	Anna Freud Centre, UK
Katarzyna Wac	University of Copenhagen, Denmark
Mads Frost	IT University of Copenhagen, Denmark
Maria Angela Ferrario	Lancaster University, UK
Maria Wolters	University of Edinburgh, UK
Mariano Alcaniz	Laboratorio de Neurotecnologías Inmersivas
Mark Matthews	University of Cornell, USA
Pedro Gamito	Universidade Lusófona, Portugal
Rosa Banos	Universidad de València, Spain
Stefano Triberti	Università Cattolica di Milano, Italy
Willem-Paul Brinkman	Delft University of Technology, The Netherlands

Contents

Psychophysiological Specificity of Four Basic Emotions Through Autobiographical Recall and Videos

Alice Chirico[1(✉)], Pietro Cipresso[1,2], and Andrea Gaggioli[1,2]

[1] Department of Psychology, Università Cattolica Del Sacro Cuore, Milan, Italy
{alice.chirico,andrea.gaggioli}@unicatt.it
[2] Applied Technology for Neuropsychology Lab, Istituto Auxologico Italiano,
IRCCS, Milan, Italy
{p.cipresso,a.gaggioli}@auxologico.it

Abstract. Current theories of emotion generally agree that basic emotions involve several systems with a considerable degree of specificity at the psychophysiological level. Analyzing the psychophysiological profiles of emotions allowed to understand if individuals felt the target emotional states or if they perceived it into the emotional material. Here, we explored the sensitivity of autobiographical recall and videos in reproducing emotional psychophysiological specificity even in the lab. We recorded 40 participants' psychophysiological profiles of anger, fear, joy, sadness elicited through videos and autobiographical recall, following a within subject design, in a counterbalanced order. We assessed the autonomic responding (i.e., heart rate) during each emotion induction (3 min length) using a ProComp Infinity 8-channel (Thought Technology Ltd, Montreal, Canada). The sampling rate was set at 256 Hz. We followed the guidelines of Task Force of the European Society of Cardiology and the North American Society of Pacing and Electrophysiology, to extract typical temporal and spectral HRV measures and to evaluate the response of the autonomic nervous system. Specifically, we classified the rhythms as very low frequency (VLF, <0.04 Hz), and high frequency (HF, 0.15 to 0.4 Hz) oscillations. Results showed that emotions induced through autobiographical recall could be better differentiated than those elicited using videos. We found significant interaction effects of 4 emotions × 2 conditions (video vs. autobiographical recall) measuring both sympathetic (VLF) and parasympathetic activity (HF). Autobiographical recall could recreate a differential activation of the sympathetic and parasympathetic nervous system for each emotion, which was mostly in line with existing literature. However, videos did not allow discriminating different emotional states clearly at the psychophysiological level. These findings suggested autobiographical recall as a more suitable technique to recreate basic emotions' psychophysiological activation in the lab. Finally, these results offered some insights into the issue of whether emotions induced in the lab are perceived or really felt by participants.

Keywords: Psychophysiology · Patterning · Basic emotions · Videos
Autobiographical recall · Emotion specificity

© ICST Institute for Computer Sciences, Social Informatics and Telecommunications Engineering 2018
P. Cipresso et al. (Eds.): MindCare 2018, LNICST 253, pp. 1–8, 2018.
https://doi.org/10.1007/978-3-030-01093-5_1

1 Introduction

Even if researchers are far from providing a consensual definition of "emotion", most of them agree that emotions are complex processes involving different systems, such as the motivational, experiential, behavioral and physiological one [1–4]. Several scholars focused on the psychophysiological activation occurring during an emotional episode and conceived it as an adaptive response triggering the best behavior to face the eliciting situation [5–8]. Given the great interest in this component, researchers have developed several perspectives to explain its role in the emotional process. One of the longest-lasting perspective concerns the extent to which the Autonomous Nervous System (ASN) could be differentially activated in different emotions (see [8–11]). In other words, this view investigates if and to what extent different emotions are characterized by differential somato-visceral activations.

Despite many controversies still exist on the extent of patterning of the ANS in emotions, several studies have shown a considerable degree of specificity regarding psychophysiological activation related to basic emotions of joy, fear, sadness and anger [9, 10, 12, 13]. With this regard, the temporal regulation of the cardiac function has resulted as a reliable measure to differentiate patterns of autonomous activity related to basic emotions with respect to a neutral stimulus, and elicited through autobiographical recall technique [14]. This measure allows for detecting both the parasympathetic and the sympathetic nervous system activation by computing R-R intervals during a continuous tachogram. Anger emerged as characterized by an increasing heart rate but little fluctuations in high frequency (HRV). Happiness, fear and sadness reported an increase of sympathetic activation but a decrease in parasympathetic activation. Fear was also characterized by co-occurrent changes in respiration, while sadness and happiness were not.

In other words, these findings evidenced that it is possible to differentiate emotions according to their psychophysiological profile. However, an open issue concerns the extent to which the emotions recalled through autobiographical recall technique could be closer to the equivalent real ones. It is widely known that memory implies a reconstruction of past events, since it is not a mere copy of them [15]. This would lead to inaccurate and less intense relived emotional experiences, even in the lab [16, 17]. To address this issue, researchers have focused also on other emotion-inducing techniques such as videos, which are able to induce real-time emotions (e.g., [18, 19]. However, the ability of these two conventional techniques (i.e., videos and autobiographical recall) to discriminate among different emotions at the psychophysiological level has to be tested yet.

This is far more relevant if considering that measuring psychophysiological profile of emotions could be a measure of the emotionally *lived* experience besides of the *reported* one. In other words, the assessment of psychophysiological profiles of emotions allowed detecting felt emotions and not only reported ones [20].

Indeed, studying emotion in real context has always been a relevant issue due to the fleeting nature of the emotional states [21]. Conversely, reproducing emotions in the lab allows controlling for their effect on other psychological processes [22], as well as for investigating hidden mechanisms underlying these phenomena (e.g., [23]).

Here, we explored the sensitivity of two conventional emotion-induction techniques (autobiographical recall and videos) to reproduce emotional psychophysiological specificity of *felt* joy, anger, fear, sadness even in the lab. This allowed also monitoring each ongoing emotional experience during its occurrence, thus focusing on the experienced emotions and not on the self-reported or perceived ones.

2 Methodology

2.1 Sample and Procedure

The study sample comprised 40 adults (21 women) volunteers from Italy. Their mean age was 20.07 (S.D. = 1.42). We chose a within-design in which each participant was exposed to joy, anger, fear, sadness inducing stimuli conveyed both through videos and autobiographical recall in a counterbalanced order. Upon arrival to the lab, participants signed formed consent, and the physiological monitoring equipment was installed. Each emotional induction and concurrent psychophysiological measurement lasted 3 min. At the end of each session, participants fixed a graphical quadrant depicting each of the four basic emotions in terms of intensity and type of emotion. This was taken as a measure of the extent to which participants felt the target emotion.

2.2 Measures and Instruments

Psychophysiological Measures. We assessed the autonomic responding (i.e., heart rate) during each emotion induction (3 min length) using a ProComp Infinity 8-channel (Thought Technology Ltd, Montreal, Canada). The sampling rate was set at 256 Hz. We followed the guidelines of Task Force of the European Society of Cardiology and the North American Society of Pacing and Electrophysiology [24], to extract typical temporal and spectral HRV measures and to evaluate the response of the autonomic nervous system. Specifically, we classified the rhythms as very low frequency (VLF, <0.04 Hz), and high frequency (HF, 0.15 to 0.4 Hz) oscillations.

Videos. According to guidelines provided by literature [25], we exposed participants to four emotional contents conveyed through videos (1 joy-inducing stimuli; 1 anger-inducing stimulus; 1 fear stimulus; 1 sadness stimulus) displayed on a LCD monitor. The joy-inducing video showed a scene from the film "*Pretty woman*". The anger-inducing video was taken from the film "*Total Recall*". The fear-inducing video displayed a scene from the film "*The ring*". The sadness-inducing video featured a scene from the film "*The pursuit of happiness*". Each video lasted 3 min (Table 1 and Fig. 1).

Table 1. The table reports the content of each video.

Stimuli	Content
Joy inducing stimulus	The final scene in which Richard Gere says, "I love you" to Julia Roberts
Anger inducing stimulus	The main character (Arnold Schwarzenegger) underwent a inevitable procedure and his anger explodes
Fear inducing stimulus	Samara (the ghost) comes out of the tv
Sadness inducing stimulus	The main character and his son shut themselves in a public toilet to sleep but someone tries to enter, thus they try to keep it closed and they cry

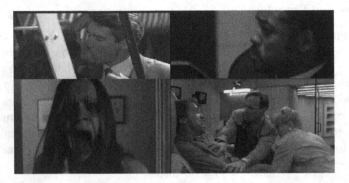

Fig. 1. The four film clips. Joy (Top-left), Sadness (top-right); Fear (bottom-left); Anger (bottom-right).

Autobiographical Recall. Participants were required to recall joyful, anger-related, fearful and sad autobiographical emotional episodes while watching at a black screen monitor with a cross at the centre of it. After, we started recording psychophysiological signals. Participants were required to close their eyes and relive the target emotion as vividly as they could while remembering the target event. We followed the same procedure described in [14].

3   Data Analysis

We carried out two separated repeated measure ANOVAs 2 (condition: autobiographical recall vs. video) × 4 (content: joy vs. anger vs. fear vs. sadness) for each of the three indexes of sympathetic (Low Frequency- LF; Very Low Frequency-VLF) and parasympathetic activation (High Frequency-HF).

4 Results

Results showed that emotions induced through autobiographical recall could be better differentiated than those elicited using videos. Specifically, we found significant interaction effects of 4 emotions $\times$ 2 conditions (video vs. autobiographical recall) measuring both sympathetic (through VLF) $[F(3,117) = 4.148; p < .01; \eta^2 = 0.096]$ and parasympathetic activity (through HF) $[F(3,117) = 3.824, p < .05; \eta^2 = .089]$ (Table 2 and Figs. 2 and 3).

Table 2. Descriptive statistics for VLF and HF for each emotion

	VLF				HF			
	Autobiographical recall		Video		Autobiographical recall		Video	
	Mean	Std. Err.	Mean	Std. Err.	Mean	Std. Err.	Mean	Std. Err.
Anger	18.45	1.33	21.94	1.56	1270.34	307.85	315.12	79.02
Fear	22.73	1.71	20.23	1.48	1017.90	213.02	288.64	73.84
Joy	24.73	1.54	21.77	1.44	545.44	100.00	241.37	47.42
Sadness	29.29	2.28	23.04	1.74	520.14	110.93	222.84	39.24

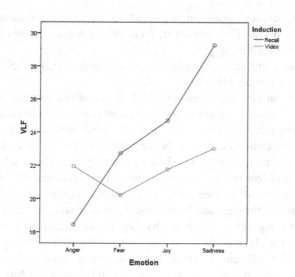

Fig. 2. Interaction effect 4 emotions $\times$ 2 conditions (video vs. autobiographical recall) measuring both sympathetic with VLF as a measure.

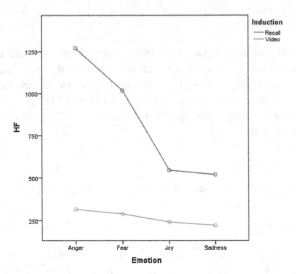

Fig. 3. Interaction effect 4 emotions × 2 conditions (video vs. autobiographical recall) measuring both sympathetic with HF as a measure.

5   Discussion and Conclusion

Emotion-induction studies relied on the need to overcome limitations related to studying emotions *in vivo* [21]. However, recreating emotional states in the lab has always been a challenge [26, 27].

Despite a wide array of emotion-induction techniques exist, their potential and limitations are still to be deeply analyzed yet.

An open issue concerns the extent to which the emotions recalled by an autobiographical technique could be closer to the equivalent real ones, compared to real-time emotions induced by means of videos. In this study, we demonstrated that videos could induce real-time emotions that can be better differentiated at a physiological level. Maybe, the reconstruction of events required by memory during a recall would lead to, at least, different, and less intense relived emotional experiences, even in the lab [16, 17]. This, in turn, would affect their psychophysiological profile. Results demonstrated that emotions induced through autobiographical recall could be better differentiated than those elicited using videos, as shown by the two significant interaction effects for VLF and HF. Specifically, (see descriptive statistics), Autobiographical recall resulted as able to recreate a differential activation of the sympathetic and parasympathetic nervous system for each emotion, which was mostly in line with existing literature [14]. However, videos did not allow to discriminate different emotional states clearly at a psychophysiological level. These findings suggested autobiographical recall as a more suitable technique to recreate basic emotions' psychophysiological activation in the lab. To address this issue, researchers have focused also on other emotion-inducing techniques such as videos, which are able to induce real-time emotions.

These results are promising regarding the adoption of a specific emotion-induction methodology in the lab. Indeed, it emerged that the differential psychophysiological activation of different emotions was reproduced. Specifically, *felt* emotions were better reproduced by means of autobiographical recall, instead of videos. Although an integrated assessment of psychophysiological measures and self-reported ones would be useful to draw conclusions regarding differences between felt and reported emotions, these results suggest that more advanced techniques should be adopted to study real-time emotions. With this regard, it would be useful to integrate peripheral measures of emotions with neural ones to obtain a more comprehensive model of how emotional processes take place, even in the lab.

All these findings help gain new knowledge about the impact of a specific emotion-induction technique on the subsequent *felt* emotional state, thus allowing for the exploration of impact on other psychological processes, such as attention, prosocial behaviors, health and well-being. One possibility is Virtual Reality [28–31] and 360° immersive videos, which proved as effective tools to induce even complex emotional states in the lab [32, 33]. Finally, psychophysiological indexes could be useful also to assess the effectiveness of emotion-regulation trainings (e.g., [34]) since they target really felt emotions.

References

1. Lewis, M., Haviland-Jones, J.M., Barrett, L.F.: Handbook of Emotions. Guilford Press, New York (2010)
2. Lerner, J.S., Keltner, D.: Fear, anger, and risk. J. Pers. Soc. Psychol. **81**(1), 146 (2001)
3. Lench, H.C., Flores, S.A., Bench, S.W.: Discrete emotions predict changes in cognition, judgment, experience, behavior, and physiology: a meta-analysis of experimental emotion elicitations. Psychol. Bull. **137**(5), 834 (2011)
4. Frijda, N.H.: Emotions and action. In: Feelings and Emotions: The Amsterdam Symposium (2004)
5. Cannon, W.B.: Bodily Changes in Pain, Hunger, Fear, and Rage: An Account of Recent Researches into the Function of Emotional Excitement. D. Appleton, New York (1916)
6. Lang, P.J.: The cognitive psychophysiology of emotion: fear and anxiety (1985)
7. Frijda, N.H.: The emotions: studies in emotion and social interaction. Edition de la (1986)
8. Stemmler, G.: Physiological processes during emotion. In: The Regulation of Emotion, pp. 33–70 (2004)
9. Levenson, R.W.: The autonomic nervous system and emotion. Emot. Rev. **6**(2), 100–112 (2014)
10. Kreibig, S.D.: Autonomic nervous system activity in emotion: a review. Biol. Psychol. **84** (3), 394–421 (2010)
11. Stemmler, G., Aue, T., Wacker, J.: Anger and fear: separable effects of emotion and motivational direction on somatovisceral responses. Int. J. Psychophysiol. **66**(2), 141–153 (2007)
12. Ekman, P., Levenson, R.W., Friesen, W.V.: Autonomic nervous system activity distinguishes among emotions. Am. Assoc. Adv. Sci. **221**, 1208–1210 (1983)
13. Adolphs, R.: The biology of fear. Curr. Biol. **23**(2), R79–R93 (2013)
14. Rainville, P., et al.: Basic emotions are associated with distinct patterns of cardiorespiratory activity. Int. J. Psychophysiol. **61**(1), 5–18 (2006)

15. Schacter, D.L.: Searching for Memory: The Brain, the Mind, and the Past. Basic Books, New York (2008)
16. Levine, L.J.: Reconstructing memory for emotions. J. Exp. Psychol. Gen. **126**(2), 165 (1997)
17. Buchanan, T.W.: Retrieval of emotional memories. Psychol. Bull. **133**(5), 761 (2007)
18. Griskevicius, V., Shiota, M.N., Neufeld, S.L.: Influence of different positive emotions on persuasion processing: a functional evolutionary approach. Emotion **10**(2), 190 (2010)
19. Parrott, W.G., Hertel, P.: Research methods in cognition and emotion. In: Handbook of Cognition and Emotion, pp. 61–81 (1999)
20. Tsuchiya, N., et al.: No-report paradigms: extracting the true neural correlates of consciousness. Trends Cogn. Sci. **19**(12), 757–770 (2015)
21. Pascual-Leone, A., Herpertz, S.C., Kramer, U.: Experimental designs and the 'emotion stimulus critique': hidden problems and potential solutions in the study of emotion. Psychopathology **49**(1), 60–68 (2016)
22. Martin, M.: On the induction of mood. Clin. Psychol. Rev. **10**(6), 669–697 (1990)
23. Carvalho, S., et al.: The emotional movie database (EMDB): a self-report and psychophysiological study. Appl. Psychophysiol. Biofeedback **37**(4), 279–294 (2012)
24. Heart rate variability: standards of measurement, physiological interpretation, and clinical use. Task force of the European society of cardiology and the North American society of pacing and electrophysiology. Circulation **93**, 1043–1065 (1996)
25. Ray, R.D., Gross, J.J.: Emotion elicitation using films. In: Coan, J.A., Allen, J.J.B. (ed.) Handbook of Emotion Elicitation and Assessment, pp. 9–28. Oxford University Press, New York (2007)
26. Gilet, A.: Procédures d'induction d'humeurs en laboratoire: une revue critique [Mood induction procedures: a critical review]. L'encéphale **34**, 233–239 (2008)
27. Westermann, R., Stahl, G., Hesse, F.: Relative effectiveness and validity of mood induction procedures: analysis. Eur. J. Soc. Psychol. **26**, 557–580 (1996)
28. Diemer, J., et al.: The impact of perception and presence on emotional reactions: a review of research in virtual reality. Front. Psychol. **6**, 26 (2015)
29. Felnhofer, A., et al.: Is virtual reality emotionally arousing? Investigating five emotion inducing virtual park scenarios. Int. J. Hum. Comput. Stud. **82**, 48–56 (2015)
30. Riva, G., et al.: Transforming experience: the potential of augmented reality and virtual reality for enhancing personal and clinical change. Front. Psychiatry **7**, 164 (2016)
31. Riva, G., et al.: Affective interactions using virtual reality: the link between presence and emotions. CyberPsychol. Behav. **10**(1), 45–56 (2007)
32. Chirico, A., Cipresso, P., Gaggioli, A.: Psychophysiological correlate of compex spherical awe stimuli. Neuropsychol. Trends (2016)
33. Chirico, A., et al.: Effectiveness of immersive videos in inducing awe: an experimental study. Sci. Rep. **7**(1), 1218 (2017)
34. Shiota, M.N., et al.: Beyond happiness: building a science of discrete positive emotions. Am. Psychol. **72**(7), 617 (2017)

Extraversion Affects Attentive Processes of Personal Images

Pietro Cipresso[1,2(✉)], Miriam Fanciullo[2], Giuseppe Riva[1,2],
and Emanuela Saita[2]

[1] Applied Technology for Neuro-Psychology Lab,
Istituto Auxologico Italiano, Milan, Italy
{p.cipresso,bepperiva}@auxologico.it,
[2] Department of Psychology, Università Cattolica del Sacro Cuore, Milan, Italy
mirifanc@libero.it,
{pietro.cipresso,giuseppe.riva,
emanuela.saita}@unicatt.it

Abstract. Personality traits are an important part of the psychology with so many study to consider this actually a huge field. On the other hand, the relationship between personality traits and attentional process has not been deepen extended yet, above all using technological advanced measures to quantify attention. In this study we selected personal and neutral photos presenting all of them to the participants while tracking the eyes movements by using an eye-tracker. Results showed that personal images have in general higher number of fixation and more saccades. Specifically, while extroverts showed no differences in exploring personal and neutral photos, introverts participants showed an higher number of fixations and more saccades for personal images than neutral. These results if confirmed in further studies pone interesting questions about the role of personality in attentional processes linked to personal experiences.

Keywords: Psychometrics · Personality · Attention · Personal images
Extraversion · Eye-tracking

1 Introduction

Photos and other images are quite simple and efficient tool to be used for induction where are proposed as stimuli for experimental psychology [1]. On the other hand the use of personal image provided directly by the participants to the experiment are very rare. One of the main problems that makes personal images not so used is that they are not able to be standard, by definition.

As empirical based science, psychology need to use standard tests that can be replicated and so used also for other studies [2]. However the chance to use personalized stimuli can be a catalyst for new ideas and indeed keen empirical science.

Personalized stimuli can be used, for example for working with episodic memory pushing both cognitive psychology and emotional science [3].

© ICST Institute for Computer Sciences, Social Informatics and Telecommunications Engineering 2018
P. Cipresso et al. (Eds.): MindCare 2018, LNICST 253, pp. 9–14, 2018.
https://doi.org/10.1007/978-3-030-01093-5_2

1.1   Toward an Integrated Approach

Since we used a personalized tool, the experimental complexity increased a lot and the risk of biases was to be taken into serious consideration.

Even if standardization of experimental stimuli remains in our opinion very crucial, there are different situations or studies, in both clinical and experimental settings, in which the enrichment of personal cues might be crucial and keen. The role of emotions and episodic memory, might be related to personal images in a very strong way [4]. Potentially these aspects could be driver of our behavior already in focus attentional process and so having an impact in decision making processes and other outcome of consequent actions [5].

Our hypothesis, in this study, was to find a preliminary evidence of a relationship between personal images and focused attention measured with eye-tracking, being this an objective and reliable instrument to catch such a sensible and fast construct such as the attention.

Moreover, we hypothesized that some personality traits were able to affect this relationship, and in particular we considered that more introvert people was prone to focus more on personal image, being them more focused on their own sphere than the social one.

2   Materials and Methods

2.1   Participants

Twenty-three students (19 females) attended the Faculty of Psychology at the Catholic University of Sacred Heart of Milan, Italy, and took part in the experiment. All the participants were students, also in psychology or communication, but without previous knowledge of eye-tracking and in particular with no knowledge of the attentional processes investigated in the experiment. Social, economic, cultural and historical background were all similar since all the participants were student in the same University and with similar background. They were first met by one of the researchers during academic courses or through personal contacts and then contacted via mail and/or telephone to schedule a meeting at the laboratory where the eye-tracker were installed. The topics associated with the experiment were not mentioned during academic courses or personally.

Two of the participants failed to complete the experimental session due to personal or technical problems and were excluded from statistical analyses. The final sample was composed of 21 students, who were assessed with the TIPI personality test [6] to be considered more or less introverts or extroverts.

2.2   Procedure

Participants where contacted months before of the experimental session and were required to provide soon after 30 personal photos mixing people and places. Xx of these photos were selected by a psychology researcher to be comparable with the neutral photos. An analysis of perceptive salience of all the photos has been done by using Matlab, in order to endure that all the stimuli were not able to grab the attention due to perceptive processes.

Researchers then created specific algorithms to include all the photos of each participants in the pipeline to be be presented to each subject as her/his own personal stimulus but mixed with the neutral photos.

Once in the laboratory the day of the experiment, the participants were required to fulfill some questionnaires. In particular the TAS-20 for alexitimia [7]; State Traits Anxiety Inventory, STAI-Y [8]; TIPI for personality [6]; and finally the Self Assessment Manikin SAM [9], for evaluating perceived level of physiological arousal, emotional valence, and dominance.

At this point the experimental task started. The participants were required to watch the monitor in front of them, staying still, while the head position was kept through an opportune hardware support for the chin. The photos were showed from the custom algorithm while the eye-movements were tracked at the same time.

2.3   Signal Acquisition and Data Analysis

The experiment was carried out in the labs, equipped with two portable PCs, one for delivering the stimuli and the other for acquiring eye-tracker data.

The pupillometry data were acquired using an Eye-link 1000, including experimental design software to record all raw signals, then exported and resampled at 1000 Hz.

In our study, by using the eye-tracker data extraction, we obtained for each participant a matrix of gaze and pupil data corresponding to each stimuli presentation (all the personal and neutral photos); in particular, we collected 1000 rows for each second (sampling to 1000 Hz), thereby making it possible to establish the exact period of each stimulus in the pipeline.

The software for the eye tracker was programmed to process the eye-movement indicators in terms of the number of fixations and saccades, that quantify the level of attention spent in each photo.

3   Results

Results have been highlighted following. In particular, we reported the descriptive statistics for both the questionnaires (Table 1) and for eye-tracking indexes (Table 2).

Within, between and interaction effects are highlighted in a 2 × 2 mixed experimental design with the *within condition* (Personal vs. Neutral) by the *between condition* TP score (extroverts vs. introverts) (Table 3).

Results showed that personal images have in general higher number of fixation and more saccades (Fig. 1). This means that participants were more prone to focus to personal images than neutral, but this was of course expected, being the photo personal. Indeed, the interesting result is the different attentional levels of introverts and extroverts. In fact, while extroverts showed no differences in exploring personal and neutral photos, introverts participants showed an higher number of fixations and more saccades for personal images than neutral (Table 2 and Fig. 1).

Table 1. Descriptive statistics for questionnaires

Measure	N	Min	Max	Mean	St. Err.	St. Dev.
STAI (state)	21	26	50	35.05	1.319	6.045
STAI (traits)	23	29	62	41.61	1.851	8.877
TAS score	23	28	58	42.39	1.851	8.877
TP score E	23	2.00	7.00	4.9130	.33216	1.592
TP score A	23	3.50	7.00	5.3913	.21769	1.043
TP score C	23	2.50	7.00	5.6522	.25814	1.237
TP score N	23	1.50	6.50	3.5652	.23587	1.131
TP score O	23	2.50	7.00	5.2609	.24726	1.185
SAM score (valence)	22	1.27	2.64	1.9008	.09456	.44351
SAM score (arousal)	22	1.55	3.64	2.4545	.12446	.58379
SAM score (dominance)	22	2.82	4.73	3.8182	.10514	.49316

Table 2. Descriptive statistics for eye-tracking indexes

Measure	Measure type	Condition	Personality	Mean	St. Dev.	N
Average duration of eye blinks	Attention	Personal photos	Introverts	108.6841	48.22675	8
			Extrovert	158.3728	32.25470	13
			Total	139.4438	45.27270	21
		Neutral photos	Introverts	157.2698	83.46548	8
			Extrovert	182.4577	62.22686	13
			Total	172.8623	70.13327	21
Number of fixations	Attention	Personal photos	Introverts	32.9205	5.18249	8
			Extrovert	30.4196	4.25359	13
			Total	31.3723	4.66957	21
		Neutral photos	Introverts	28.9217	3.00181	8
			Extrovert	29.4030	3.74981	13
			Total	29.2196	3.41288	21
Number of saccades	Attention	Personal photos	Introverts	32.2614	5.29361	8
			Extrovert	29.6783	4.29180	13
			Total	30.6623	4.74465	21
		Neutral photos	Introverts	28.2912	3.09526	8
			Extrovert	28.6119	3.77153	13
			Total	28.4897	3.45158	21
Mean pupil dilation	Emotional intensity	Personal photos	Introverts	1,052.3041	258.35748	8
			Extrovert	940.8391	304.43339	13
			Total	983.3019	286.43734	21
		Neutral photos	Introverts	1,045.7377	303.52697	8
			Extrovert	919.8932	269.47547	13
			Total	967.8340	282.37695	21

Table 3. Univariated tests for eye-tracking indexes

Experimental condition	Measure	F	Sig.	Partial Eta²
Condition (*within factor*)	Average duration of eye blinks	10.514	*.004*	.356
	Number of fixations	12.301	*.002*	.393
	Number of saccades	12.188	*.002*	.391
	Mean pupil dilation	.548	.468	.028
Condition X TP score entroversion/extraversion (*interaction*)	Average duration of eye blinks	1.195	.288	.059
	Number of fixations	4.349	*.051*	.186
	Number of saccades	4.051	*.059*	.176
	Mean pupil dilation	.150	.703	.008
TP score entroversion/extraversion (*between factors*)	Average duration of eye blinks	2.620	.121	.122
	Number of fixations	.355	.558	.018
	Number of saccades	.432	.519	.022
	Mean pupil dilation	.874	.362	.044

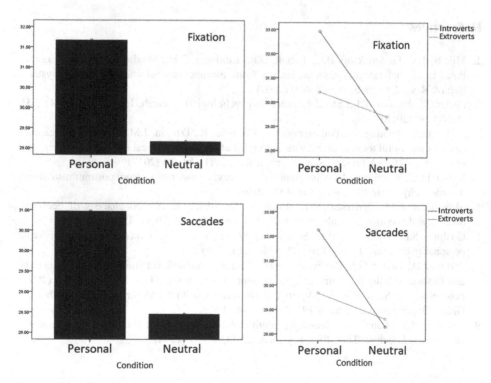

Fig. 1. Fixation and saccades in both personal and neutral photos for both introverts and extroverts.

This indicates that the difference between personal and neutral images is mostly due to the contribution of introverts that tends to focus significantly more than extroverts when they focus on personal images than neutral.

4 Discussion

With this preliminary study we were interested in understanding (1) if personal images were related to attentional processes, and (2) if personality traits, and in particular more introvert people, were more focused on their own personal images that others.

Results showed that the relationship between personal images and attentional processes is crucial, but the extend to which this can be considered so strong to have an effect is still to be verified in further studies.

On the other hand, we faced statistical differences in the attention that introverts dedicated to personal images, where extroverts showed no differences. The results are still too preliminary to draft any conclusions but the effects that, once verified, this could have on the field is really interesting and deserve to be discussed and explored in further works, even exploiting other aspects of personality and also focusing on the whole spectrum of the personality traits than in two opposite extreme.

References

1. Mikels, J.A., Frederickson, B.L., Larkin, G.R., Lindberg, C.M., Maglio, S.J., Reuter-Lorenz, P.A.: Emotional category data on images from the international affective picture system. Behav. Res. Methods 5(4), 626–630 (2007)
2. Fisher, R., Milfont, T.L.: Standardization in psychological research. Int. J. Psychol. Res. 31 (1), 88–96 (2010)
3. Allé, M.C., Manning, L., Potheegadoo, J., Coutelle, R., Danion, J.M., Berna, F.: Wearable cameras are useful tools to investigate and remediate autobiographical memory impairment: a systematic PRISMA review. Neuropsychol. Rev. 27(1), 81–99 (2017)
4. Rubin, D.C.: Emotion and autobiographical memory: considerations from posttraumatic stress disorder. Phys. Life Rev. 7(1), 132–133 (2010)
5. Mowincke, A.M., Pedersen, M.L., Eilertsen, E., Biele, G.: A meta-analysis of decision-making and attention in adults with ADHD. J Atten. Disord. 19(5), 355–367 (2015)
6. Gosling, S.D., Rentfrow, P.J., Swann Jr., W.B.: A very brief measure of the big five personality domains. J. Res. Pers. 37, 504–528 (2003)
7. Parker, J.D., Taylor, G.J., Bagby, R.M.: The 20-item toronto alexithymia scale: III. Reliability and factorial validity in a community population. J. Psychosoma Res. 55(3), 269–275 (2003)
8. Pedrabissi, L., Santinello, M.: Verifica della validità dello STAI forma Y di Spielberger. Giunti Organizzazioni Speciali 191–192, 11–14 (1989)
9. Bradley, M.M., Lang, P.J.: Measuring emotion: the self-assessment manikin and the semantic differential. J. Behav. Ther. Exp. Psychiatr. 25(1), 49–59 (1994)

A "First Look" on Frailty: A Scientometric Analysis

Elisa Pedroli[1(✉)], Pietro Cipresso[1,2], Silvia Serino[1,2],
Desirèe Colombo[1,3], Michelle Semonella[1], Andrea Gaggioli[1,2],
and Giuseppe Riva[1,2]

[1] Applied Technology for Neuro-Psychology Lab,
IRCCS Istituto Auxologico Italiano, Via L. Ariosto 13, 20145 Milan, MI, Italy
{e.pedroli,p.cipresso,s.serino}@auxologico.it,
semonellamichelle@gmail.com
[2] Department of Psychology, Catholic University, Largo Gemelli 1, 20100
Milan, MI, Italy
{pietro.cipresso,silvia.serino,
giuseppe.riva}@unicatt.it
[3] Department of Basic Psychology, Clinic and Psychobiology, Universitat
Jaume I, Av. Sos Baynat, s/n, 12071 Castelló de la Plana, Castellón, Spain
dcolombo@uji.es

Abstract. Frailty is a new and interesting concept that describes a preclinical condition in which elderly are more vulnerable and the possibility to develop pathologies increases. Often, the physical decline is related to cognitive impairments: Subjects in this situation are defined as cognitive frail patients. The literature connected to this syndrome is growing steadily and a bibliometric analysis is needed to better understand the evolution and the current state of the art. In this article, several domains are analyzed: Authors, categories, countries, institutions and journals. An interesting scenario emerged from the data: On the one hand, outcomes show a strong interest in understanding the real diffusion of this phenomenon using demographics and statistical methods. On the other hand, it emerged the increasing application of mathematical models to the study of medical phenomena.

Keywords: Frailty · Scientometric · Bibliometric · Cognitive frailty

1 Introduction

Ageing is a physiological process involving both cognitive and motor domains, and affecting therefore many aspects of everyday life. According to the World Health Organization, the proportion of people older than 60 years-old is increasing rapidly and faster than all the other age groups [1]. Within this part of the population, in the last decade there has been a lot of interest in "frail" patients, constituting the 6.9% of adults older than 65-year-old [2]. Specifically, frailty is a clinical condition and a state of vulnerability associated with increasing age and affecting multiple domains like gait, mobility, balance and cognition [3]. According to the standardized definition of Fried and colleagues, three or more of the following criteria should be met: Unintentional weight loss (10 lbs in past year), self-reported exhaustion, weakness (grip strength), slow walking speed, and low physical activity [2]. This condition has been directly associated with higher risks for adverse health outcomes, such as mortality, disability and, especially, high risk of falls [2, 4–6]. A few years after the systematization of this concept, the International Consensus Group organized by the International Academy on Nutrition and Ageing (IANA) and the International Association of Gerontology and Geriatrics (IAGG) proposed the identification of a new important condition: "Cognitive frailty" [7]. This new definition is strongly connected with physical frailty, but it also requires the presence of cognitive impairments in addition to the criteria mentioned above, whereby, the main factors of cognitive frailty are: (1) Presence of physical frailty and cognitive impairments, and (2) exclusion of concurrent dementia or underlying neurological conditions [7, 8]. In order to diagnose cognitive frailty, a complete neuropsychological assessment is needed [8]. However, a specific profile has not yet been clearly defined: As a consequence, some authors describe cognitive frailty as a hypothetical condition without clear available data to support it. However, this construct is potentially interesting as it would allow to identify a promising target condition for the development of preventive interventions against age-related problems, with a main focus on the rehabilitation of both cognitive and physical aspects.

It is well known that chronic diseases may accelerate ageing through a reduction of the body's adaptation abilities. Decreased physiological reserve leads to a homeostatic imbalance or frailty, a pre-clinical condition that increases the possibility to developed pathologies [9]. Therefore, a timely intervention could lead to a great advantage and to a better healthy outcome. A rehabilitation programs will must be focused on both physical and cognitive aspects.

Even though cognitive and motor impairments have been always considered and treated independently, literature is showing evidence for a strong relation between them, both in healthy and pathological conditions. An example of this relationship is the risk of falls. Among frail patients, indeed, falls are one of the most critical public health problems, as well as the major cause of injuries: One in three old people, indeed, falls at least once in a year [10], with subsequent consequences in terms of loss of independence and adverse psychosocial problems [11, 12].

In this article, we present a systematic and computational analysis of the state of the art of the frailty field in terms of various co-citation networks, aiming at exploring the evolution of the intellectual structure of this knowledge domain over time.

2 Methods

Data Collection. The input data for the analyses were retrieved from the scientific database Web of Science Core Collection, based on a topic search for Frailty papers published during the whole timespan covered. The data were lastly updated on October 11, 2017. Web of Science Core Collection is composed of: Citation Indexes, Science Citation Index Expanded (SCI-EXPANDED) –1970-present, Social Sciences Citation Index (SSCI) –1970-present, Arts & Humanities Citation Index (A&HCI) –1975-present, Conference Proceedings Citation Index- Science (CPCI-S) –1990-present, Conference Proceedings Citation Index- Social Science & Humanities (CPCI-SSH) –1990-present, Book Citation Index– Science (BKCI-S) –2009-present, Book Citation Index– Social Sciences & Humanities (BKCI-SSH) –2009-present, Emerging Sources Citation Index (ESCI) –2015-present, Chemical Indexes, Current Chemical Reactions (CCR-EXPANDED) –2009-present (Includes Institut National de la Propriete Industrielle structure data back to 1840), Index Chemicus (IC) –2009-present. The resultant dataset contained a total of 11,071 records. The bibliographic records contained various fields, such as author, title, abstract, and all the references (needed for the citation analysis). The research tool to visualize the networks was Cite space v.4.0.R5 SE (32 bit) 32 under Java Runtime v.8 update 91 (build 1.8.0_91-b15). Statistical analyses were conducted using Stata MP-Parallel Edition, Release 14.0, StataCorp LP.

3 Results

The analysis of the literature on frailty shows a complex panorama. Here we will try to systematize this field in order to understand how literature has developed both temporally and geographically, which are the major areas of interest and who are the most productive authors.

3.1 Authors

Articles Counts. The top ranked author by article count is Rockwood K, with a total of 235 articles. The second one is Walston JD, with an article count of 139. The third is Morley JE, with an article count of 121. The 4th is Fried LP, with an article count of 121. The 5th is Vellas B with an article count of 107. The 6th is Mitnitski A with an article count of 107. The 7th is Cesari M with an article count of 101. The 8th is Ferrucci L with an article count of 85. The 9th is Hubbard RE with an article count of 66. The data are reported in Fig. 1.

The picture clearly shows that Rockwood, Mitnitski, and Hubbard are strongly interconnected among them, as well as Fried, Ferrucci, Walston, Vellas, and Cesari.

18   E. Pedroli et al.

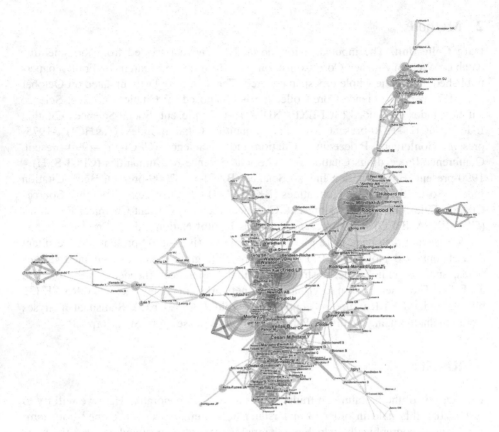

Fig. 1. Network of authors: the dimension of the nodes represents centrality.

3.2 Categories

Articles Counts. The top ranked journal by article count is GERIATRICS & GERONTOLOGY with a total of 3599 articles. The second one is GERONTOLOGY with an article count of 1895. The third is MATHEMATICS with an article count of 1033. The 4th is MEDICINE with an article count of 1025. The 5th is STATISTICS & PROBABILITY with an article count of 998. The 6th is GENERAL & INTERNAL MEDICINE with an article count of 881. The 7th is CARDIOVASCULAR SYSTEM & CARDIOLOGY with an article count of 789. The 8th is CARDIAC & CARDIOVASCULAR SYSTEMS with an article count of 685. The 9th is PUBLIC with an article count of 650. The 10th is SURGERY with an article count of 604. A graphical representation of this analysis is reported in Fig. 2.

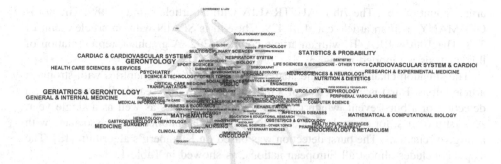

Fig. 2. Network of categories. The dimension of the nodes represents centrality

3.3 Countries

Articles Counts. The top ranked country by article count is USA with a total of 3732 articles. The second one is ENGLAND with an article count of 874. The third is CANADA with an article count of 824. The 4th is ITALY with an article count of 636. The 5th is FRANCE with an article count of 603. The 6th is NETHERLANDS with an

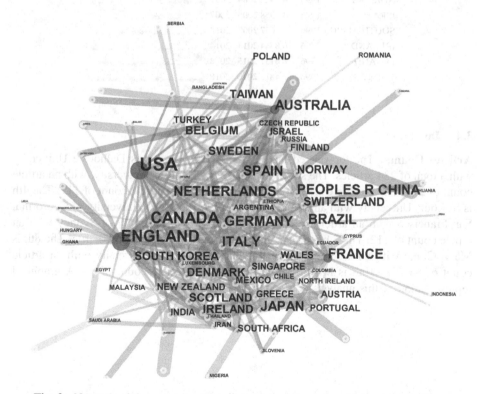

Fig. 3. Network of the countries. The dimension of the nodes represents centrality.

article count of 569. The 7th is AUSTRALIA with an article count of 489. The 8th is GERMANY with an article count of 429. The 9th is SPAIN with an article count of 398. The 10th is BRAZIL with an article count of 292. A graphical representation of this analysis is reported in Fig. 3.

The situation changes when the analysis is focused on the countries with strongest article bursts. Burst is an indicator of a most active area of research. Burst represent a detection of a burst event, which can last for multiple years as well as a single year. A burst provides, for example, evidence that a particular publication is associated with a surge of citations. The burst detection was based on Kleinberg's algorithm [13]. The Top 11 includes almost all European nations, as showed in Table 1.

Table 1. Top 11 countries with strongest citation bursts.

Countries	Year	Strength	Begin	End	1996 - 2018
USA	1996	7.8515	1996	1997	
DENMARK	1996	15.9834	1997	2006	
ENGLAND	1996	3.7486	1998	1999	
FINLAND	1996	3.2681	1998	2004	
SWEDEN	1996	5.0102	2002	2004	
NORWAY	1996	4.9469	2004	2007	
ISRAEL	1996	3.4958	2005	2007	
SOUTH AFRICA	1996	4.3657	2007	2013	
IRELAND	1996	10.8544	2013	2014	
POLAND	1996	8.6131	2015	2018	
TURKEY	1996	3.4813	2015	2018	

3.4   Institutions

Articles Counts. The top ranked institution by article count is Dalhousie University with a total of 234 articles. The second one is Johns Hopkins University, with an article count of 213. The third is University of Michigan with an article count of 117. The 4th is St Louis University with an article count of 114. The 5th is University of California, San Francisco with an article count of 113. The 6th is University of Sydney with an article count of 112. The 7th is Duke University with an article count of 105. The 8th is Mayo Clinic with an article count of 92. The 9th is Yale University with an article count of 84. The 10th is McGill University with an article count of 84. A graphical representation of this analysis is reported in Fig. 4.

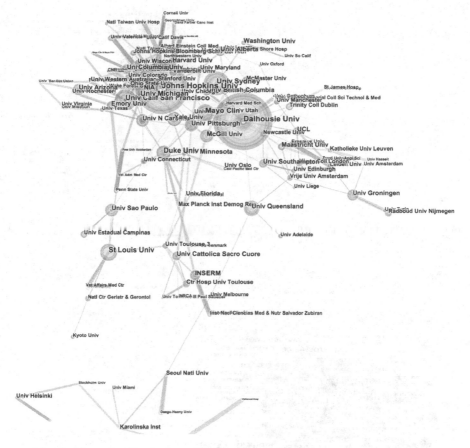

Fig. 4. Network of institutions. The dimension of the nodes represents centrality.

3.5   Journals

Citations Counts. The top ranked journal by citation count is JOURNAL OF THE AMERICAN GERIATRICS SOCIETY with a total of 5058 citations. The second one is THE JOURNAL OF GERONTOLOGY, SERIES A: BIOLOGICAL SCIENCES AND MEDICAL SCIENCES with a citation count of 5040. The third is JAMA-JOURNAL OF THE AMERICAN MEDICAL ASSOCIATION with a citation count of 3042. The 4th is NEW ENGLAND JOURNAL OF MEDICINE with a citation count of 2965. The 5th is AGE AND AGEING with a citation count of 2847. The 6th is LANCET with a citation count of 2795. The 7th is ARCHIVES OF INTERNAL MEDICINE with a citation count of 2189. The 8th JOURNAL OF NUTRITION HEALTH & AGEING with a citation count of 1682. The 9th is JOURNAL OF THE AMERICAN MEDICAL DIRECTORS ASSOCIATION with a citation count of 1554. The 10th is BRITISH MEDICAL JOURNAL with a citation count of 1509. A graphical representation of this analysis is reported in Fig. 5.

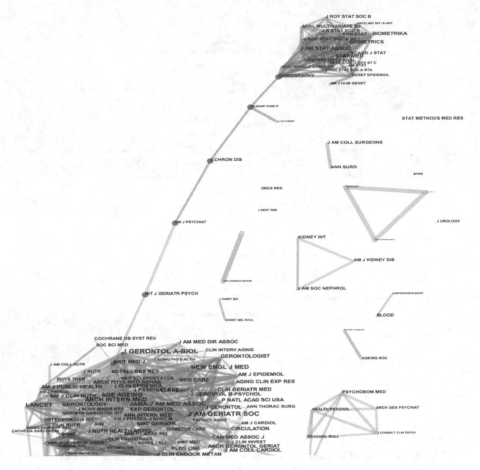

Fig. 5. Network of Journals: The dimension of the nodes represents centrality.

4 Discussion

In order to understand the complex panorama of frailty literature, we analyzed the data from Web of Science using scientometrics techniques. The factors included in this analysis are: authors, categories, countries, institutions and journals. An interesting scenario emerged from the data.

Concerning the "Categories" section, it is not surprising to find "GERIATRICS & GERONTOLOGY", and "GERONTOLOGY" at the top of the list. Interestingly, the third and fifth positions are occupied by "MATHEMATICS", and "STATISTICS & PROBABILITY". This trend highlights two important factors. On the one hand, it shows a strong interest in understanding the real diffusion of this phenomenon using demographics and statistical methods. On the other hand, these outcomes highlight the increasing application of mathematical models to the study of medical phenomena.

The analysis involving the count of articles per country show that the observed network is well connected, and it includes 6 European and 4 non-European countries. This data chances analyzing the countries with strongest citation bursts. Table 1 highlights that, to the current literature, the interest in frailty is moving from the USA to European nations; specifically, Denmark and Ireland are leading the top positions for article burst.

Another particular result emerged from the analysis of journals. As showed in Fig. 5, two different clusters of journals that deal with frailty emerged: The bigger one is related to medical and health topics. The second and smaller one is about biostatistics and epidemiologic. These outcomes relate to what emerged from the Categories' analysis and stress the strong interest that is emerging in the use of statistical and mathematical models for the understanding and prediction of frailty.

These analyses are a "first look" at this phenomenon, but a future deeper study is needed to better clarify the situation and the new trend in the study of frailty.

Acknowledgments. The article was supported by the Italian funded project "High-end and Low-End Virtual Reality Systems for the Rehabilitation of Frailty in the Elderly" (PE-2013-02355948).

References

1. Woollacott, M., Shumway-Cook, A.: Attention and the control of posture and gait: a review of an emerging area of research. Gait Posture **16**(1), 1–14 (2002)
2. Fried, L.P., et al.: Frailty in older adults: evidence for a phenotype. J. Gerontol. A Biol. Sci. Med. Sci. **56**(3), M146–M156 (2001)
3. Gobbens, R.J., et al.: Toward a conceptual definition of frail community dwelling older people. Nurs. Outlook **58**(2), 76–86 (2010)
4. Speechley, M., Tinetti, M.: Falls and injuries in frail and vigorous community elderly persons. J. Am. Geriatr. Soc. **39**(1), 46–52 (1991)
5. Fried, L.P., et al.: Untangling the concepts of disability, frailty, and comorbidity: implications for improved targeting and care. J. Gerontol. A Biol. Sci. Med. Sci. **59**(3), 255–263 (2004)
6. Rockwood, K.: What would make a definition of frailty successful? Age Ageing **34**(5), 432–434 (2005)
7. Kelaiditi, E., et al.: Cognitive frailty: rational and definition from an (IANA/IAGG) international consensus group. J. Nutr. Health Ageing **17**(9), 72–734 (2013)
8. Delrieu, J., et al.: Neuropsychological profile of "cognitive frailty" subjects in MAPT study. J. Prev. Alzheimer's Dis. **3**(3), 151 (2016)
9. Panza, F., et al.: Cognitive Frailty: A Potential Target for Secondary Prevention of Dementia. Taylor & Francis, Milton Park (2017)
10. Blake, A.J., et al.: Falls by elderly people at home: prevalence and associated factors. Age Ageing **17**(6), 365–372 (1988)
11. Donald, I.P., Bulpitt, C.J.: The prognosis of falls in elderly people living at home. Age Ageing **28**(2), 121–125 (1999)
12. Zijlstra, G.A., et al.: Prevalence and correlates of fear of falling, and associated avoidance of activity in the general population of community-living older people. Age Ageing **36**(3), 304–309 (2007)
13. Kleinberg, J.: Bursty and hierarchical structure in streams. Data Min. Knowl. Discov. **7**(4), 373–397 (2003)

Using an Aging Simulator Suit for Modeling Visuo-Motor Limitations of Elderly Users Interacting with a Mobile Application: Feasibility Study

Andrea Gaggioli[1,3(⊠)], Chiara Settimi[2], Pietro Cipresso[1,3],
Elisa Pedroli[3], Marco Stramba-Badiale[3], and Giuseppe Riva[1,3]

[1] Department of Psychology, Università Cattolica del Sacro Cuore, Milan, Italy
{andrea.gaggioli, pietro.cipresso,
giuseppe.riva}@unicatt.it
[2] Università Cattolica del Sacro Cuore, Milan, Italy
[3] I.R.C.C.S. Istituto Auxologico Italiano, Milan, Italy
{andrea.gaggioli, p.cipresso, stramba_badiale,
giuseppe.riva}@auxologico.it

Abstract. With the rapid ageing of the population, designing inclusive mobile interfaces that match accessibility requirements is an important challenge. Here, we report results of an exploratory study, which investigated the feasibility of using an "aging simulator suit" for modeling the sensorimotor limitations of elderly users interacting with a tablet application. The study involved one experimental group ("simulated ageing" condition, SA) and two normative comparison groups ("elderly control" condition, EA; and "young control" condition, YC). In the SA condition, a group of young adults (N = 60; mean age = 26.1, s.d. = 4.0) carried out a visuo-motor task while wearing the aging simulator suit, which reproduced three levels of visuo-motor impairment: (i) visual; (ii) motor; (iii) visual and motor. In the EC condition, the same visuo-motor task was executed by a sample of healthy elderly individuals (N = 20; mean age = 73.5, s.d. = 6.3). In the "young control" (YC) condition, the task was executed by a sample of young adults (N = 40; mean age = 24.6; s.d. = 4.7). Results showed that accuracy and speed of YC outperformed performance of EC and SA. Furthermore, SA approximated EC performance, suggesting that aging simulator suit may provide a reliable model of visuo-motor limitations of the normative-aged group. Implications of these findings for design practice are discussed.

Keywords: Inclusive design · Accessibility · Aging simulator suit
Visuo-motor limitation · Mobile applications

1 Introduction

According to a recent UN report [1], in the next fifteen years, the number of people in the world aged 60 years or over is projected to grow to 1.4 billion, reaching nearly 2.1 billion by 2050. As the senior population progressively increases, it will also increase the proportion of elderly individuals using mobile and ubiquitous computing devices.

P. Cipresso et al. (Eds.): MindCare 2018, LNICST 253, pp. 24–33, 2018.
https://doi.org/10.1007/978-3-030-01093-5_4

Therefore, designing universally accessible mobile applications has become an important challenge to address in order to ensure that elderly individuals can exploit the full range of opportunities offered by the mobile digital revolution. In this context, the concept of accessibility refers to the discriminatory aspects related to equivalent user experience for people with disabilities, including people with age-related impairments [2]. A key requirement for improving the accessibility of products is to put the user at the center of the design process, which is the core principle of the so-called "universal design". According to Christophersen [3], universal design involves three knowledge processes: (i) user-designer interaction: any tool or technique that designers apply in order to align the requirements of the end-user with the characteristics of the product; (ii) understanding people: to collect information that allows deepening the under-standing of the target user group (including i.e., range of abilities, potential impair-ments, contextual factors etc.); (iii) evidence-based findings: to analyze previous experiences (both positive and negative) of existing products to inform the design of future products. Within the context of universal design, a significant challenge concerns how to create reliable and informative model of end user abilities, which is even more relevant when dealing with elderly users interacting with mobile applications. User modeling has a significant role in enhancing the accessibility of user interfaces since it allows defining them by taking into consideration the needs and eventual limitations of the target. Here, we report results of an exploratory study, which investigated the feasibility of using an "aging simulator suit" as a new approach for modeling the sensorimotor limitations of elderly users interacting with a mobile device application. Aging simulators are wearable devices that are designed to generate embodied models of physical and sensorial limitations of an elderly individual. These tools have been applied in education and health disciplines [4] while their use in universal design is still very limited. Specifically, our research examined the effects of ageing simulator on sensorimotor performance of young adult participants under three different simulated impairment levels (visual, motor, and visuo-motor), using two simple visuo-motor coordination tasks, which participants were asked to execute as quickly and accurate as possible on a tablet device. Performance in this experimental condition was contrasted with two control conditions: a normative elderly group; and a young adults group, who executed the same tasks without wearing the ageing suit.

2 Method

2.1 Participants

All participants involved in the study were unpaid volunteers. Informed consent was obtained after the nature of the procedures had been fully explained. In overall, the study involved 120 participants, of which 100 young adults and 20 healthy elderly individuals. Young adults participants were included in the study if they matched the following inclusion criteria: age $\geq$ 21 years; normal vision or corrected-to-normal with glasses or contact lenses; absence of motor impairments on the dominant hand. Elderly adults participants were included in the study if they matched the following inclusion criteria: age $\geq$ 65 years; age-related (expected) decline of vision loss, or near-normal vision (in the better eye, with best possible glasses correction); age-related (expected) decline of bimanual and uni-manual motor skills. Exclusion criteria included: abnormal vision changes caused by disorders of the visual system; evidence of medical, neurologic, or psychiatric conditions that could adversely affect motor function; evidence of cognitive impairment (Mini-Mental Status Examination cut-score of 24 or below). A test of hand dominance was performed on all participants. Summary statistics for demographic variables across conditions are shown in Tables 1 and 2.

Table 1. Descriptive statistics for demographic variables across conditions

Condition	N	F	M	Mean age	S.D.
EC	20	10	10	73.050	6.2616
YC	40	20	20	24.575	4.7116
SA-V	20	10	10	27.450	4.2361
SA-M	20	10	10	24.600	3.7892
SA-VM	20	10	10	26.250	3.9719
Total	120	60	60	33.417	18.4166

SA = simulated ageing group (overall); SA-V: simulated ageing group (visual impairment); SA-M: simulated ageing group (motor impairment) SA-VM simulated ageing group (visual and motor impairment).

Table 2. Descriptive statistics for hand dominance across conditions

Condition	Right	Left	Total
EC	20	0	20
YC	35	5	40
SA-V	19	1	20
SA-M	17	3	20
SA-VM	20	0	20
Total	111	9	120

SA = simulated ageing group (overall); SA-V: simulated ageing group (visual impairment); SA-M: simulated ageing group (motor impairment) SA-VM simulated ageing group (visual and motor impairment).

2.2   Apparatus and Materials

2.2.1   Aging Simulator Suit

The GERT aging simulator suit [5] (Fig. 1) includes several components, which can be used either alone, or in combination in order to make the user experiencing the sensorimotor limitations of older persons.

Since the present study focused on the modeling of visuo-motor coordination ability in interacting with a tablet-based app, only the functionalities of the GERT suit that could potentially interfere with this ability were selected; more specifically, the impairments selected were:

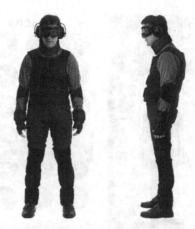

Fig. 1. The GERT ageing simulation suit used in this study.

- opacity of the eye lens and narrowing of the visual field (caused by the special glasses);
- head mobility restrictions (caused by the cervical collar);
- restricted joint mobility (caused by the elbow wraps);
- sinking strength and changed coordination (caused by the weight cuffs);
- restricted grip ability and reduced tactile perception (caused by the special gloves).

Young adults participants assigned to the SA-V condition worn the special glasses only; participants assigned to the SA-M condition worn only the components of the GERT that were expected to cause limitations of the motor function in the upper limb and torso; finally, participants assigned to the SA-VM condition performed the tasks wearing both the special glasses and the components of the GEAR suit that limited the motor function in the upper limb and torso.

2.2.2 Tablet Applications Used for the Visuo-Motor Tasks

The mobile device used to perform the visuo-motor task was an Apple iPad 2. The task was performed on two commercial applications available on the Apple Store: "Finger Balance" e "Tap the Dots". The first application challenges the player with a fine motor coordination task, consisting in balancing a ball on a rod. Task difficulty can be gradually increased during the gameplay, i.e., by changing the inclination of the rod. The "Tap the Dots" application requires the player to tap as many buttons as possible within 60 s. The target button flashes within a grid, in a random way. Game configuration options allow setting the task difficulty by increasing or decreasing the speed of the gameplay.

For both applications, users' performance was assessed in terms of speed and accuracy, following the arrangement outlined in Table 3.

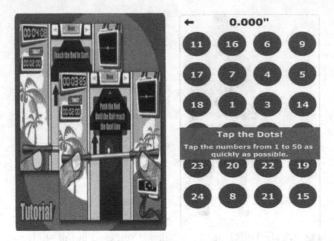

Fig. 2. Screenshots of the tablet applications selected to implement the visuo-motor tasks. Left: the Finger Balance application; Right: the Tap the Dots application.

Table 3. Structure of visuo-motor tasks and performance measures

Application	Difficult levels	Number of trials for each level	Total number of trials	Performance measures
Finger Balance	5	3	15	Task completion time (sec) and number of errors
Tap the Dots	1	3	3	Task completion time (sec) and number of correct choices

2.3   Procedure

Participants signed the informed consent and filled the demographic questionnaires. Next, they received the experimental instructions: participants were explained the two games and asked to be fast and accurate in solving the tasks. After the briefing, the experimenter assisted participants in the SA condition in dressing the components of the GERT age simulator suit and provided them with safety guidelines. Next, participants were given the iPad tablet with the pre-installed applications to begin the experiment. The order of the tasks performed with the two applications was counterbalanced across participants at each condition. The overall experimental procedure lasted about 35–40 min for each participant.

3   Data Analysis and Results

All participants successfully completed the experimental procedures. Data were analysed by mean of statistical software package IBM SPSS Statistics v. 21. We first performed a correlation analysis of accuracy and speed variables across selected tasks. Results of correlation analysis on performance variables is reported in Table 4.

Table 4. Correlation analysis of accuracy and speed variables across selected tasks

		FB	FB	T+	T+
		Mean errors	Mean total time	Mean hits	Mean response time
FB	Pearson correlation	1	.417**	−.407**	.598**
Mean errors	Sig. (2-tailed)		.000	.000	.000
	N	120	120	120	120
FB	Pearson correlation	.417**	1	−.387**	.340**
Mean total time	Sig. (2-tailed)	.000		.000	.000
	N	120	120	120	120
T+	Pearson correlation	−.407**	−.387**	1	−.652**
Mean hits	Sig. (2-tailed)	.000	.000		.000
	N	120	120	120	120
T+	Pearson correlation	.598**	.540**	−.652**	1
Mean response time	Sig. (2-tailed)	.000	.000	.000	
	N	120	120	120	120

FB = *Finger Balance* application; T+: *Tap the Dots* application
*p < 0.05 and **p < 0.01

As predictable, accuracy and speed measures were positively correlated within each task. Furthermore, a positive correlation was found between measures of accuracy and speed across the two different tasks. This finding suggests that the selected tasks provided an independent, but related measure of participants' visuo-motor performance.

Two repeated-measures ANOVA were carried out to determine the effects of condition type (EC, YC, SA-V, SA-M and SA-VM) on accuracy of task execution and time (see also Table 3). The first ANOVA was carried out on the Finger Balance task data. Condition served as a between-subjects factor and trial repetition (3 levels) and degree of difficulty (5 levels) served as within-subject factor. The second ANOVA was carried out on the Tap the Dots task data; again, condition type served as a between-subjects factor, and trial repetition (3) served as within-subject factor.

3.1   Results of Repeated ANOVA for Finger Balance Task

Results showed a significant effect of condition on number of errors ($F_{(4; 115)} = 21.791$, $p < 0.01$). Post-hoc comparisons were carried out using Bonferroni adjustment for correcting the significance level, showing that the EC group made significantly more errors than each of the other conditions; none of the remaining contrasts were significant.

The effect of condition on response time was also significant ($F_{(4; 115)} = 19.422$, $p < 0.01$). Post-hoc contrasts revealed that the EC group was significantly slower than

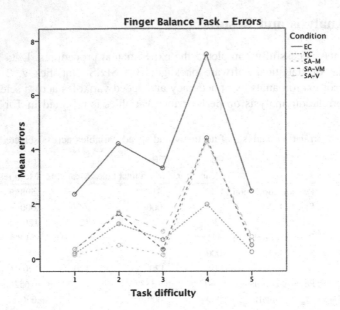

Fig. 3. Mean errors for each experimental condition, on five increasing task difficulty levels (Finger Balance task).

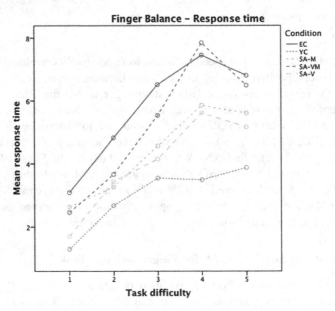

Fig. 4. Mean time response for each experimental condition, on five increasing task difficulty levels (Finger Balance task).

each of the other conditions, with the exception of SA-VM. The following graphs depict mean errors (Fig. 2) and time (Fig. 3) for each experimental condition, on five increasing task difficulty levels.

3.2 Results of Repeated ANOVA for Tap the Dots Application

Results of the second repeated ANOVA showed a significant effect of condition on number of target hits ($F_{(4; 115)} = 21.791$, $p < 0.01$). Post-hoc comparisons (with Bonferroni adjustment) revealed that the EC group hit significantly less targets than the remaining conditions. In addition, the YC condition produced significantly more hits than SA-VM, which was also significantly less accurate than SA-V and SA-M (see Fig. 4).

ANOVA conducted on response time for Tap the Dots application showed a significant effect of condition on response time $F_{(4; 115)} = 44.432$, $p < 0.01$). Post-hoc contrasts showed that the EC group was significantly slower than each of the other conditions, while the YC condition performed significantly faster than SA-VM. In addition, the SA-VM condition was significantly faster that EC but also significantly slower than SA-V, SA-M and YC (see Figs. 5 and 6).

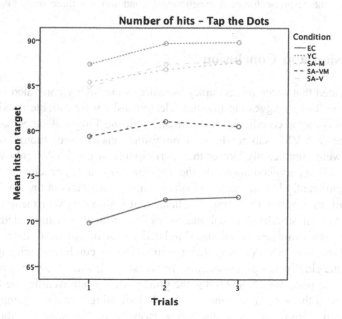

Fig. 5. Mean hits on target for each experimental condition, on three consecutive trials (Tap the Dots application).

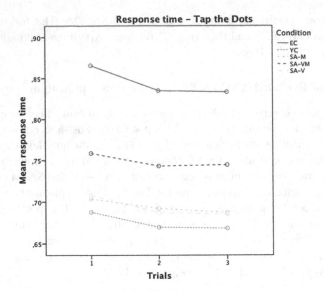

Fig. 6. Mean time response for each experimental condition, on three trials (Tap the Dots application).

4 Discussion and Conclusion

Results indicated that speed and accuracy measures were highly correlated within each task and across tasks, suggesting that the selected tasks were reliable proxies of participants' visuo-motor coordination performance. In the Finger Balance task, participants in the SA-VM sub-condition (combining visual and motor impairment simulation) were significantly slower than participants in the SA-V (only visual) and SA-M (only motor) sub-conditions. In the Tap the Dots task, participants in the SA-VM were significantly less accurate and slower than participants in the SA-V and SA-M sub-conditions. Overall, these results indicate that within the experimental condition, the combination of simulated visual and motor impairment was more detrimental to performance than simulated visual and simulated motor impairment alone. Results of the repeated measure ANOVA revealed a main effect of condition indicating that, as predictable, the elderly group performed at the worst level, while the young adult group performed at the best level. Noteworthy, the young adult group wearing the GERT suit performed on both tasks at intermediate level, indicating that the ageing simulator decreased their visuo-motor coordination performance. Furthermore, the post-hoc contrasts revealed that for both tasks, the combination of simulated visual and motor impairment determined the best approximation of the performance of the normative elderly group, indicating that the visual and motor modules of the GERT had an additive detrimental effect on users' speed and accuracy. Overall, these preliminary findings suggest that the ageing simulator suit could be used to model, at least in an approximate order, the effects of age-related visuo-motor impairments on interactive tasks involving mobile applications. The "first-person" experience of sensory and physical challenges associated with aging generated by the GERT (or by devices alike) could help designers in gaining a better understanding of these limitations and provide them with new insights concerning the development of more inclusive and accessible user interfaces. Furthermore, the age simulation suit could be potentially used for carrying out preliminary usability tests to evaluate perceptual and motor issues of users' accessibility in mobile interfaces for older people.

Acknowledgments. This work was partially supported by the MIUR grant CTN01-00128-297089 Design4All and by the MDS grant Frail-VR (PE-2013-02355948).

References

1. United Nations: Department of Economic and Social Affairs, Population Division. World Population Ageing (2015)
2. Web Accessibility Initiative: Accessibility, Usability, and Inclusion: Related Aspects of a Web for All. https://www.w3.org/WAI/intro/usable. Accessed 15 Sept 2017
3. Christophersen, J. (ed.): Universal Design: 17 Ways of Thinking and Teaching. Husbanken, Norway (2002)
4. Cannon-Diehl, M.R., Rugari, S.M., Jones, T.S.: High-fidelity simulation for continuing education in nurse anesthesia. AANA J. **80**(3), 191–196 (2012)
5. http://www.age-simulation-suit.com/ Accessed 15 Sept 2017

The Italian Adaptation of Interpersonal Communication Competences Questionnaire

Michelle Semonella[1], Alice Chirico[2(✉)], Elisa Pedroli[1],
Andrea Gaggioli[1,2], and Giuseppe Riva[1,2]

[1] Applied Technology for Neuropsychology Lab, Istituto Auxologico Italiano,
IRCCS, Milan, Italy
semonellamichelle@gmail.com, e.pedroli@auxologico.it
[2] Department of Psychology, Università Cattolica del Sacro Cuore, Milan, Italy
{alice.chirico, andrea.gaggioli, a.gaggioli,
giuseppe.riva, bepperiva}@unicatt.it

Abstract. There has been a growing interest in assessing interpersonal communication competences, to understand how to empower them in specific domains. The aim of this study was to create an Italian adaptation of the Interpersonal Communication Competence Scale (ICCS), by Rubin & Martin. The study was designed to assess the structure of the ICCS and to determine the number of components needed to adequately describe the psychological constructs of Interpersonal Communication Competence in the Italian sample. The questionnaire was administered to 137 subjects. Adopting an analytic process using an exploratory factor analysis, the steps yield a seven factor solution composed of 26 items. We discussed results and future directions concerning interpersonal communication competence scale.

Keywords: Interpersonal communication competences · Questionnaire
ICCS · Psychometrics · Italian adaptation · Communication

1 Introduction

Interpersonal communication skills can be conceived as the ability to (i) communicate intentions and information in an assertive way within a communication setting, (ii) to manage and control the surrounding environment, (iii) to disclose to others, and (iv) to stand up for own rights [1]. These competences are an essential part of people' daily life in several social and cultural contexts, e.g., work, family and significant interpersonal relationships [2], since they deserve to accomplish one's relevant goals, such as obtaining information, gaining support, and exchanging ideas and opinions [3]. Finally, these abilities can help people improve their relationship in terms of empathy, support, comprehension and control.

© ICST Institute for Computer Sciences, Social Informatics and Telecommunications Engineering 2018
P. Cipresso et al. (Eds.): MindCare 2018, LNICST 253, pp. 34–41, 2018.
https://doi.org/10.1007/978-3-030-01093-5_5

Given the relevance of these skills, there has been a growing interest in assessing interpersonal communication competences, to understand how to empower them in specific domains such as adult-infant relationship [4], work, and hospital setting [5].

However, there is still a need of a tool able to assess the general cross-domain dimensions of interpersonal communication skills. Moreover, a general communication competence scale in Italian has not been developed yet. We have reviewed different questionnaires in other languages [6], and at the end of the process the Interpersonal Communication Competence Scale of Rubin & Martin [7], has been selected in order to be adapted into Italian.

First, the ICCS is quick and easy to administer, counting 30 items (24 positive and 6 reverse code), with a high internal consistency (Global Cronbach Alpha = .86), and covering cross-domain interpersonal communication skills. Specifically, ICCS is based on 10 cross-domain dimensions of Interpersonal Communication concerning individuals' capability to manage communication in interpersonal settings [7]: (i) self-disclosure is the capability to open ourselves to others [8]; (ii) empathy concerns an affective component resounding with others and a cognitive one, which entails taking others' perspective [9]; (iii) social relaxation concerns feeling comfortable during a conversation [5]; (iv) assertiveness, is the capability of individuals to show their emotions, opinions and to stand up for their rights [7]; (v) interaction management, as the ability to manage everyday interactions [10]; (vi) altercentrism, the capability to put others – and not ourselves - under the spotlight [11]; (vii) expressiveness, regards to be frank during a conversation both verbally and verbally [12]; (viii) supportiveness, a way to communicate that is descriptive, provisional, spontaneous, oriented towards solving problem, empathic and egalitarian [1]; (ix) immediacy, the capability to show others that are willing for communication [13]; and (x) environmental control, is the ability to control the communication setting [14].

These 10 dimensions correspond to akin personal skills and social skills, which are inter-related in a complex way. Therefore, identifying specific cross-domain sub-factors can be crucial for future studies interested in how different cognitive, emotional and social skills contribute to an improvement in communication competences.

Starting from these premises, this study aimed at adapting the Interpersonal Communication Competence Scale in an Italian sample.

2   Methodology

2.1   Sample and Procedure

The Italian version of the ICCS questionnaire was administered to 137 adults (86 women) volunteers from Italy (males mean age = 29.71; S.D. = 7.209; females mean age = 25.96; S.D. = 5.675) recruited through a snowball sampling (online announcements and flyers). Mean schooling of Males was 18 years (S.D. = 5.185), mean schooling of females was 16.75 (S.D. = 2.588). Participants were required to complete the online version of the ICCS questionnaire along with socio-demographic questions using Qualtrics platform (https://www.qualtrics.com/it/).

2.2 Measures and Instruments

The Italian ICCS version was a translation of the original questionnaire, with exactly alike item numbering. First, two bilingual translators (one expert in the field of emotions and the other naïve) translated ICCS into the Italian, as suggested by [15]. Further, the goodness of translation was tested by a back version from Italian to English, done by two bilingual other translators, both fluent in Italian and English. The back-translation was checked by one of the authors of the original version. Afterwards, the original and back versions were compared to define the final Italian form by three expert judges.

Participants were required to complete the questionnaire following this response scale: "If you ALMOST ALWAYS interact in this way, select 5; "If you communicate this way OFTEN, select 4"; "If you communicate this way SOMETIMES, select 3"; "If you act this way only SELDOM, select 2"; "If you ALMOST NEVER behave in this way, select 1".

Table 1 reports item of the Italian version.

Table 1. The table reports items of the full Italian version of the ICCS.

Original	Italian
1. I allow friends to see who I really am	1. Lascio che gli amici vedano chi sono veramente
2. Other people know what I am thinking	2. Le altre persone capiscono ciò che sto pensando
3. I reveal how I feel to others	3. Mostro agli altri come mi sento
4. I can put myself in others' shoes	4. Riesco a mettermi nei panni degli altri
5. I don't know exactly what others are feeling (R)	5. Non riconosco accuratamente le emozioni altrui
6. Other people think that I understand them	6. Le altre persone pensano che io li capisca
7. I feel comfortable in social situations	7. Mi sento a mio agio nei contesti sociali
8. I feel relaxed in a small group gatherings	8. Mi sento rilassato in un gruppo di poche persone
9. I feel insecure in groups of strangers. (R)[a]	9. Mi sento insicuro in un gruppo di persone che non conosco
10. When I've been wronged, I confront the person who wronged me	10. Quando subisco un torto, affronto la persona che ne è l'artefice
11. I have troubles standing up for myself. (R)	11. Ho problemi a farmi valere
12. I stand up for my rights	12. Difendo i miei diritti
13. My conversations are pretty one-sided. (R)	13. Le mie conversazioni sono abbastanza unilaterali
14. I let other know that I understand what they say	14. Faccio capire agli altri che ho compreso cos'hanno detto
15. My mind wanders during conversations	15. La mia mente divaga durante le conversazioni

(continued)

Table 1. (*continued*)

Original	Italian
16. My conversations are characterized by smooth shifts from one topic to the next	16. Durante una conversazione riesco a cambiare argomento in modo fluente
17. I take charge of conversations I'm in by negotiating what topics we talk about	17. Conduco la conversazione gestendo gli argomenti di cui trattare
18. In conversations with friends, I perceive not only what they say but what they don't say	18. Durante le conversazioni con gliamici, sono in grado di cogliere non solociò che dicono, ma anche ciò che nondicono
19. My friends can tell when I'm happy or sad	19. I miei amici capiscono quando sono felice o triste
20. It's difficult to find the right words to express myself. (R)	20. Ho difficoltà nel trovare le giuste parole per esprimermi
21. I express myself well verbally	21. Mi esprimo bene verbalmente
22. My communication is usually descriptive, not evaluative	22. La mia comunicazione è di solito descrittiva, non critica
23. I communicate with others as though they're equals	23. Comunico con gli altri senza sentirmi superiore o inferiore
24. Others would describe me as warm	24. Gli altri mi descriverebbero come una persona cordiale
25. My friends truly believe that I care about them	25. I miei amici credono sinceramente che io tenga a loro
26. I try to look others in the eye when I speak with them	26. Cerco di guardare gli altri negli occhi quando parlo con loro
27. I tell people when I feel close to them	27. Confido alle persone quando sono legato a loro
28. I accomplish my communication goals	28. Raggiungo i miei obiettivi comunicativi
29. I can persuade others to my position	29. Riesco a persuadere gli altri della mia opinione
30. I have trouble convincing others to do what I want them to do. (R)	30. Ho problemi a convincere gli altri a fare quello che vorrei loro facessero

[a]R = reverse item.

3 Data Analysis

This study was designed to assess the structure of the ICCS and to determine the number of components needed to adequately describe the psychological constructs of Interpersonal Communication Competence in the Italian sample.

To this aim, a parallel Monte Carlo simulation analysis was run on the 30 items, to determine the number of factors to retain in EFA using IBM SPSS Statistics software (Version 21, release 21.0.0.0 64 bit edition). More, an EFA analysis on the original set of items was carried out. Data were analyzed by IBM SPSS Statistics software (Version 21, release 21.0.0.0 64 bit edition). No missing values were found.

4   Results

Preliminary correlations among items showed that items were from moderately to highly correlated. Results of parallel Monte Carlo simulation analysis suggested a border seven-factor solution. Given the 10 factors original structure of the scale, initially, we opted for the 7 factors solution. Both the Kaiser-Meyer-Olkin Measure of Sampling Adequacy (.802) and Bartlett's test of Sphericity [$\chi2$ (703) = 1807.91; p < .01] indicated the factoriability of the correlation matrix [16]. We carried out an exploratory factorial analysis. Principal axis factoring (PFA) and a Varimax rotation forcing a seven factor solution were used. The seven factor solution accounted for 51.886% of global variance, with each factor correlating low with other factors. Only item 10 loaded on the fourth factor, therefore, we chose to delete it, and run again PFA with Varimax rotation. This solution explained a higher proportion of variance (51.65%). However, item 15 showed the lowest level of communality (.177) and loaded low in each factor. We chose to delete it. The proportion of explained variance increased (53.169%). Item 22 showed the lowest level of communality (.261), therefore, we deleted it and run again a PFA with varimax rotation. The proportion of explained variance increased (54.271%). We retained this as the final solution (Fig. 1).

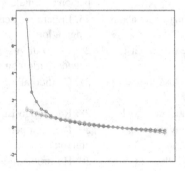

Fig. 1. Scree plot comparing PAF eigenvalues with PA eigenvalues. Dotted green line represents the random 95th percentile of PA eigenvalues and the dotted blue line represents eigenvalues from the research data. PAF = principal axis factoring analysis; PA = parallel analysis. (Color figure online)

The Scale revealed a high internal consistency (Cronbach alpha = .90) (Table 2).
Factor 1 showed a good internal consistency (.80); Factor 2 (.82); Factor 3 (.28); Factor 4 (.80); Factor 5 (.70); Factor 6 (.70); Factor 7 (.41). However, if we removed item 30 from factor 3, internal consistency increased (.66). Therefore, we computed again Cronbach alpha analysis on all items, excluding item 30, and we found that internal consistency did not change (.90). In sum, the final scale excluded items: 10;15;22;30 of the original scale.

Table 2. Factor loadings from the rotated solution of the exploratory factor analysis with varimax rotation in the final version of the scale (30 items, N = 137). Items loading for each factor were reported in bold.

Item	Factors						
	Conversation management	Social-disclosure	Social-confidence	Assertiveness	Social-closeness	Social Reax	Conversation inability
1.	.168	**.579**	.170	.033	.249	.258	−.133
2.	−.029	**.702**	.105	.018	.165	.071	.077
3.	.095	**.805**	.012	−.019	−.008	.077	−.001
4.	**.551**	.220	−.055	.058	.053	−.033	−.482
5.	−.212	−.116	−.120	−.042	.011	.076	**.559**
6.	**.619**	−.001	.094	−.001	.210	.012	−.087
7.	.285	.279	.307	.104	.135	**.707**	−.047
8.	.355	.178	−.068	−.006	.293	**.459**	−.077
9.	.091	−.118	**−.339**	−.271	.083	−.532	.042
11.	−.095	−.069	**−.763**	−.104	−.013	−.175	.238
12.	.320	.187	**.380**	−.099	.059	.100	−.113
13.	.064	.066	−.073	−.033	−.130	−.165	**.488**
14.	**.620**	.139	−.131	.088	.169	.169	−.071
16.	**.586**	−.001	.406	.223	.124	.129	.198
17.	.438	.234	**.434**	.205	−.039	.174	.315
18.	**.664**	−.010	.300	.041	−.033	−.013	−.118
19.	.004	**.648**	.027	.019	.170	.069	.022
20.	.016	.009	−.213	**−.842**	−.006	−.141	.121
21.	.427	.107	.101	**.754**	.137	.057	.006
23	.149	.314	−.073	.212	**.379**	.239	−.312
24.	.111	.321	−.193	−.027	**.556**	.100	−.132
25.	.270	.316	.194	.081	**.709**	−.028	−.017
26.	**.317**	.203	.207	.194	.316	.181	−.093
27.	.146	**.604**	.088	.087	.101	.021	−.178
28.	.453	.332	**.422**	.187	.050	.151	−.075
29.	**.456**	.040	.451	.270	.128	.148	.064
30.	−.057	−.038	**−.709**	−.118	.036	−.018	.011

5 Discussion and Conclusion

Interpersonal communication competences are the ability to express ourselves in the process of exchanging information, in a dual or group conversation, thus managing the surrounding environment, and understanding and interpreting the Other, both verbally and non-verbally [7].

Despite the relevance of considering these competences jointly in a cross-domain perspective, only few instruments have been developed, in order to investigate them [2]. After having reviewed the literature on this topic, we selected the ICCS [7] to be adapted into Italian.

We administered the questionnaire to 137 subjects. Adopting an analytic process using an exploratory factor analysis, the steps yield a seven factor solution composed of 26 items.

Factor 1: Conversation Management, is the capability to understand the explicit and the implicit level of a conversation, thus orienting it according to our communicative intentions (items: 4; 6; 14; 16; 18; 26; 29).

Factor 2: Social – **disclosure,** is the ability to let others access ourselves transparently, when we feel enough close to them (items: 1; 2; 3; 19; 27).

Factor 3: Social – **confidence,** is the ability to manage topic inside a conversation setting, standing up for our rights (items: 9; 11; 12; 17; 28).

Factor 4: Assertiveness, is the ability of a person to express himself and his thoughts, respecting others and not denying them (items: 20; 21).

Factor 5: Social- **closeness,** is the ability to recognize to other as present inside the conversation (items: 23; 24; 25).

Factor 6: Social – **relaxation,** feeling at ease during social interactions (items: 7; 8).

Factor 7: Egocentrism, to locate ourselves under the spotlight (items: 5; 13).

Internal consistency ranged between low (.41) to optimal alpha coefficients (.90). Results showed that ICCS can be considered as a strong potential tool measure interpersonal communication competences for two reasons. It is easy and quick to administer, and it is composed by several number of dimensions. Considering the α in each domain, we do not recommend the use of domains as subscales. However, future studies need to further investigate which of these skills could be the most effective driver for new interventions aimed at improving personal capabilities.

One of the main aspects that emerged from interpersonal communication was the dual dimension concerning self-expression, and others-understanding. This can be due to the fact that communication does not only consist in giving information, but it entails also understanding other's intentions [17]. This process includes a verbal and not verbal level. Communication management requires capabilities in terms of empathy, self-regulations, assertiveness in order to understand own and other emotions, and regulate them due to the circumstances [18]. Indeed, the ability to manage the conversation and the interaction inside the communication setting requires a good level of empathy and self-disclosure [19]. Therefore, future studies could deepen the role of the emotional dimension, at a social and individual level, in relation to communication skills. This could be a promising future step to investigate to what extent emotional self-regulation could impact on subsequent communication management abilities, to create evidence-based trainings promoting these skills.

Finally, despite the potential of this study for the Italian population, some limitations exist. First, we considered only a small sample. Therefore, other studies should enlarge it considering a wider sample size. Then, we focused on people with a high level of education. This aspect should be deepened by future studies to elucidate its impact on communication competences. Finally, evaluating cross-domain communication competences could be a key asset for schools, in order to detect early impairment or issues, or it could become a self-assessed tool to help people monitor their abilities, thus improving them, according to a self-empowerment perspective.

References

1. Bochner, A.P., Kelly, C.W.: Interpersonal competence: rationale, philosophy, and implementation of a conceptual framework (1974)
2. DeVito, J.A.: The Interpersonal Communication Book. Pearson, London (2015)
3. Burleson, B.R., Metts, S., Kirch, M.W.: Communication in Close Relationships. Close Relationships: A Sourcebook, pp. 245–258 (2000)
4. Anders, S.L., Tucker, J.S.: Adult attachment style, interpersonal communication competence, and social support. Pers. Relationsh. 7(4), 379–389 (2000)
5. Duran, R.L.: Communicative adaptability: a measure of social communicative competence. Commun. Q. 31(4), 320–326 (1983)
6. Spitzberg, B.H., Methods of interpersonal skill assessment. In: Handbook of Communication and Social Interaction Skills, pp. 93–134 (2003)
7. Rubin, R.B., Martin, M.M.: Development of a measure of interpersonal communication competence. Commun. Res. Rep. 11(1), 33–44 (1994)
8. Jourard, S.M.: Self-disclosure: An Experimental Analysis of the Transparent Self (1971)
9. Redmond, M.V.: The relationship between perceived communication competence and perceived empathy. Commun. Monograph. 52(4), 377–382 (1985)
10. Clark, R.A., Delia, J.G.: Topoi and rhetorical competence. Q. J. Speech 65(2), 187–206 (1979)
11. Cegala, D.J.: Interaction involvement: a cognitive dimension of communicative competence. Commun. Educ. 30(2), 109–121 (1981)
12. Bienvenu, M.J.: An interpersonal communication inventory. J. Commun. 21(4), 381–388 (1971)
13. Wiemann, J.M.: Explication and test of a model of communicative competence. Hum. Commun. Res. 3(3), 195–213 (1977)
14. Brandt, D.R.: On linking social performance with social competence: Some relations between communicative style and attributions of interpersonal attractiveness and effectiveness. Hum. Commun. Res. 5(3), 223–226 (1979)
15. Borsa, J.C., Damásio, B.F., Bandeira, D.R.: Cross-cultural adaptation and validation of psychological instruments: Some considerations. Paidéia (Ribeirão Preto) 22(53), 423–432 (2012)
16. Kaiser, H.F.: An index of factorial simplicity. Psychometrika 39(1), 31–36 (1974)
17. Grice, H.P.: Meaning. Philos. Rev. 66(3), 377–388 (1957)
18. Mayer, J.D., Geher, G.: Emotional intelligence and the identification of emotion. Intelligence 22(2), 89–113 (1996)
19. Haynes, L.A., Avery, A.W.: Training adolescents in self-disclosure and empathy skills. J. Couns. Psychol. 26(6), 526 (1979)

iStim. A New Portable Device for Interoceptive Stimulation

Daniele Di Lernia[1]([✉]) [iD], Giuseppe Riva[1,2], and Pietro Cipresso[1,2]

[1] Department of Psychology, Università Cattolica del Sacro Cuore, Largo
Gemelli, 1, 20100 Milan, Italy
{daniele.dilernia,giuseppe.riva}@unicatt.it
[2] Applied Technology for Neuro-Psychology Lab, IRCCS Istituto Auxologico
Italiano, Via Magnasco, 2, 20149 Milan, Italy
p.cipresso@auxologico.it

Abstract. The sense of the physiological condition of the entire organism (i.e. interoception) represents a fundamental perception that serves a correct and balanced functioning of the human body. Interoceptive information constitutes a core element in a variety of psycho-physiological systems and processes; therefore the possibility to consistently stimulate the interoceptive system with specifically targeted inputs has a fundamental value both in assessing and clinical settings. The article illustrates a new technological portable device able to delivered precise interoceptive parasympathetic stimuli to C-T afferents connected to the lamina I spinothalamocortical system. Interoceptive stimuli can be programmed in a variety of parameters, ranging from continuous stimulation to modulation of frequency and variance. Implications and possible applications are discussed in both assessing protocols and clinical treatments as well.

Keywords: Interoception · Interoceptive stimulation · C-Touch
C-fibers · Affective touch

1 Introduction

Interoception represents an emerging and promising topic in Neuroscience. Interoceptive perceptions can be defined as the sense of the physiological status of the entire organism [1] and they encompass a broad range of relevant biological functions that serve conscious and unconscious processes.

The central component of the interoceptive system is the anterior insular cortex (AIC) that receives information through a vast network of small un-myelinated fibers connected to the Lamina I spinothalamocortical pathway. These specific fibers, called C-Fibers compose a poly-modal afferent system that innervates the entire organism and report a wide range of inputs such as: hunger, thirst, pain, itch, temperature [2], muscle contraction [3, 4], hormonal and immune activity, cardiorespiratory function [1, 5], along with a specific type of tactile perception called C-Touch [6]. These inputs are processed in the interoceptive matrix that creates a metarepresentation of the organism's active processes also according to an explicit lateralization of the cortex. Specifically, the left and the right insula are usually coactive in the interoceptive system

P. Cipresso et al. (Eds.): MindCare 2018, LNICST 253, pp. 42–49, 2018.
https://doi.org/10.1007/978-3-030-01093-5_6

nonetheless, parasympathetic inputs are preferentially processed by the left insula [7] while sympathetic ones are usually processed by the right one [1, 8]. In the last decade, interoception emerged as a promising field of study due to the relevant meaning that interoceptive information has to the functioning of the organism. Recent evidence identified interoceptive altered processes in a broad range of clinical condition such as chronic pain [9], eating disorders [10–13], anxiety [14, 15], depression [16–20], addictions [21, 22], post-traumatic stress disorder [23], insomnia [24] and several others conditions [25, 26]. However, a primary limitation in the study of interoceptive system is the ontological difficulty to access and reproduce specific interoceptive stimuli. Albeit it is quite easy to activate pain and temperature inputs, other interoceptive stimuli (e.g. hunger, thirst, visceral sensations) are quite difficult to reproduce in a controlled manner, prejudicing the possibility to consistently explore different aspects of the interoceptive system in controlled settings. Moreover, easily reproducible interoceptive input, such as pain and temperature, are generally processed by the right insula [27, 28] due to their sympathetic high valence, leaving the whole system of parasympathetic input vastly unexplored.

Parasympathetic interoceptive input has been recently discovered as a promising research field. Among these kind of stimuli, C-Touch (or affective touch) is arguably the most interesting parasympathetic interoceptive input. C-Touch afferent fibers constitute a secondary touch system with a deep involvement in different psychophysiological pathways [29]. A prominent theory suggested their fundamental role in social contact and emotional bonding [30], moreover recent evidence demonstrated that interoceptive C-Touch can modulate body ownership and embodiment [31]. Additionally, several clinical conditions demonstrated altered perception connected to C-T afferents, suggesting implication of interoceptive touch also in psychopathological functioning [32].

Several experimental devices [31, 33–35] actually exist and are able to delivered interoceptive C-Tactile stimulation. Nonetheless, these instruments suffer from several limitations. Specifically, they are usually unable to deliver continuous stimulation and they are not able to modify the frequency and the variance of the stimuli. Moreover they usually require a fixed setup, limiting the portability of the instrument in different settings (i.e. hospitals, laboratories) and the possibility to apply stimuli to different body parts of the subject. To address these issues, the paper proposes a new technological portable device specifically designed to deliver tactile interoceptive stimuli, allowing continuous stimulation to any chosen body site along with the ability to program variance and frequency of the delivered stimuli.

2 Technical Development

The interoceptive stimulator has been designed and developed to provide continuous C-Tactile stimuli with a programmable pattern of stimulation. To pursuit this goal, the device has been designed taking in consideration all the relevant factors connected to C-T afferent fibres.

C-T fibres constitute a secondary touch system with very peculiar characteristics. They are uniquely found in not glabrous skin where they distinctively respond to light touch with a force under 2.5 mN [36, 37] and a stroking velocity between 1 and 10 cm/s [31, 38] with a mean peak of activation around 3 cm/s. Moreover they exhibit a tendency to fatigue [6, 39] and a specific after discharge pattern with a delayed acceleration effect [36, 40]. Considering these factors, the device (Fig. 1) uses a step motor, a driver, and an ARDUINO NANO as main programmable controller to deliver targeted interoceptive C-Tactile stimuli.

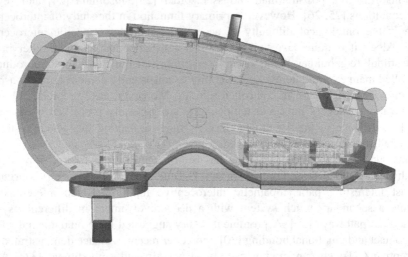

Fig. 1. Interoceptive portable stimulator with 3D printed case and calibrated probe mounted.

A LCD and a digital encoder allow selecting pre-programmed stimulation patterns directly on the device. A rechargeable battery connected to a DC Boost ensures different lines to power the step motor (12 v) and the main electronics (3 v–5 v). The device is enclosed in a specific 3D printed case that allows portability and manoeuvrability. A specifically designed and calibrated probe is attached to the step motor main shaft, providing tactile stimulation. The probe moves in circular pattern, with a linear component handled by the operator. Mixing circular and linear stimulation (Fig. 2), the probe matches the maximal mean firing frequency of CT afferents (3 cm/s ± 0.5 cm/s) [33] allowing continuous stimulation with a specific pre-calibrated force < 2.5 mN that is the optimal threshold for interoceptive touch [36, 41, 42]. Lastly, the probe oval shaped area matches the receptive CT human afferent patch ($\approx$35 mm^2) [39, 43] ensuring a targeted interoceptive stimulus.

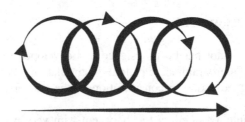

Fig. 2. Pattern of stimulation with circular and linear components.

Moreover, C-Tactile afferents show a specific behaviour of fatigue and inexcitability [6, 39] reducing their firing rate to 0 after 5 s of continuous stimulation [43], therefore the device factored several patterns of stimulation for optimal continuous performance. Mixing linear and circular stimulation, considering probe dimension, optimal velocity, and angular motion, the device fires a single CT afferent patch only for 0.28 s within a single revolution, allowing continuous stimulation without inhibition of the receptive CT field.

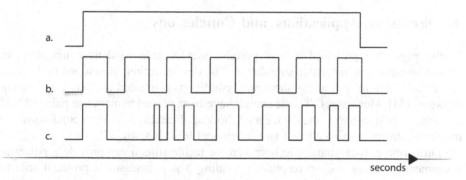

Fig. 3. Examples of programmable stimulation. (a.) continuous stimulation (b.) low variance stimulation (c.) high variance stimulation

The device is programmed with ARDUINO IDE native language. It uses common open source libraries for the digital encoder and the LCD screen. A custom library for the stepper motor driver has been developed to reduce motor time activation; the shaft can therefore reach a specific angular velocity within only 10 ms, providing almost instantaneous interoceptive stimulation in the optimal CT firing range.

The code can be updated via USB and specific stimulation patterns can be uploaded in the memory of the device and selected through the digital encoder and the LCD. The device stores stimulation patterns as STRING variables in the PROGMEM allowing the microcontroller to maintain memory also without power. A set of parameters can be controlled, such as: velocity, duration of stimulation, and pattern of stimuli. These parameters can be mixed together creating different types of interoceptive parasympathetic stimulation with various purposes.

In continuous mode (Fig. 3a) the devices activates a continuous interoceptive stimulus. Duration of the stimulation can be programmed and stored in flash memory or the device can be stopped at the appropriate time via a coded command selected through the digital encoder.

In variance stimulation (Fig. 3b and c) a predetermined pattern of stimuli with defined optimal velocity and durations is programmed in the device and selected thought the digital encoder. If selected the devices activates a series of stimuli in a fixed sequence that can be customized either for the duration of a single stimulus, the duration of the pause between stimuli, or both. Sequences can be therefore either programmed to deliver a low variance stimulation (Fig. 3b) where the device presents interoceptive stimuli with a predictable pattern; or the device can be programmed to deliver high variance stimulation, presenting a pattern of stimulation with a low predictability. Possible application of these to kind of stimulation will be presented in the discussion section.

Lastly, the device implements a SPI port that allows synchronization of stimuli between clone interoceptive stimulators in a MASTER-INDEPENDENT SLAVES configuration up to 256 devices, or in a DAISY CHAIN configuration for a larger number of cloned devices.

3   Discussion, Applications, and Conclusions

In the paper we presented a new portable device able to deliver interoceptive parasympathetic programmable stimulation. The device, entirely developed by D.D.L., has already been used to assess subclinical conditions connected to anxiety and eating disorders [44]. Moreover, C-Tactile stimuli have been proved to modulate pain [43, 45] and anxiety [43], therefore the device may show applicability in clinical conditions that require treatment both on clinical and subclinical level [44, 46, 47].

Furthermore, parasympathetic interoceptive tactile stimuli can provide a powerful instrument to assess body perception, providing a new assessment protocol able to explore the role of the body inner perceptions in different conditions.

Specifically, coactive processes in the right and left insula can be used as behavioral indexes of sympathetic and parasympathetic balance. A theoretical protocol that asks the subject to estimate the parameters of a CT parasympathetic stimulus (i.e. duration in seconds) can investigate distortions in bodily perception, indicating the presence of an alteration in the processing of the information arising from the body. In more details, according to Craig [8] a dominance of sympathetic stimuli (i.e. pain, anxiety, etc.) should distort the perception of CT stimuli duration, which should be perceived longer than real. Conversely, clinical conditions that are connected to low bodily information processing (i.e. depression, anorexia nervosa) should produce distortions in perception of CT stimuli in an opposite direction. This information might therefore be used to probe body perception and body perceptive distortions in clinical and healthy subjects.

Lastly, the device allows a complete control upon several key variables. It can be therefore programmed to deliver low or high variance stimulation with specified learning rate curves. Different variance stimulation with programmed learning rate curves has been implemented as a method to promote neuroplasticity in several applications [48]. The device might therefore utilize the same rationale to promote or suppress neuroplasticity in the interoceptive matrix. This kind of application can be theoretically applied to a variety of clinical conditions. Specifically, chronic pain, addictions, PTSD, and insomnia present hyper-activation in the cortical areas linked to the interoceptive matrix [23, 24, 26–28, 49], therefore a low variance stimulation able to reduce neuroplasticity might reduce the processing of sympathetic high arousal interoceptive stimuli in the right insula, improving clinical conditions and decreasing symptoms severity.

Conversely, a high variance stimulation aimed at enhancing interoceptive neuroplasticity can provide application in those conditions that are characterized by a low processing of bodily sensations and a functional and structural reduction of the interoceptive cortical areas, such as depression [16–19], anorexia nervosa and other eating related disorders [10–12].

Lastly, the device can also be used in complementary manner along with other technologies such as virtual reality (VR) [50], sonoception [51], and "positive technologies" [52] on a general level. For example, it can be used to improve embodiment and body ownership [31] in VR environments for clinical and assessing purposes, to modulate specific interoceptive patterns for treatments [50], or to provide interoceptive stimulation during a variety of other contexts as well (i.e. exposure therapy). These examples summarize some of the possibilities of the interoceptive stimulator, nonetheless promising evidence in the field of interoception suggests that other practical applications might be developed in future.

Author Contributions
Conceptualization, D.D.L.; Writing – Original Draft, D.D.L; Writing – Review & Editing, G.R., and P.C.; Hardware and software development: D.D.L.; Supervision G.R., and P.C.

References

1. Craig, A.D.: Interoception: the sense of the physiological condition of the body. Curr. Opin. Neurobiol. **13**(4), 500–505 (2003)
2. Cervero, F., Janig, W.: Visceral nociceptors: a new world order? Trends Neurosci. **15**(10), 374–378 (1992)
3. Mense, S., Meyer, H.: Different types of slowly conducting afferent units in cat skeletal muscle and tendon. J Physiol. **363**, 403–417 (1985)
4. Wilson, L.B., Andrew, D., Craig, A.D.: Activation of spinobulbar lamina I neurons by static muscle contraction. J. Neurophysiol. **87**(3), 1641–1645 (2002)
5. Craig, A.D.: How do you feel? Interoception: the sense of the physiological condition of the body. Nat. Rev. Neurosci. **3**(8), 655–666 (2002)
6. Iggo, A.: Cutaneous mechanoreceptors with afferent C fibres. J Physiol. **152**, 337–353 (1960)
7. Gordon, I., et al.: Brain mechanisms for processing affective touch. Hum. Brain Mapp. **34**(4), 914–922 (2013)
8. Craig, A.D.: Emotional moments across time: a possible neural basis for time perception in the anterior insula. Philos. Trans. R. Soc. Lond. Ser. B, Biol. Sci. **364**(1525), 1933–1942 (2009)
9. Di Lernia, D., Serino, S., Riva, G.: Pain in the body. Altered interoception in chronic pain conditions: a systematic review. Neurosci. Biobehav. Rev. **71**, 328–341 (2016)
10. Gaudio, S., et al.: Altered resting state functional connectivity of anterior cingulate cortex in drug naive adolescents at the earliest stages of Anorexia Nervosa. Sci. Rep. **5**, 10818 (2015)
11. Gaudio, S., et al.: White matter abnormalities in treatment-naive adolescents at the earliest stages of Anorexia Nervosa: a diffusion tensor imaging study. Psychiatry Res. **266**, 138–145 (2017)
12. Kerr, K.L., et al.: Altered insula activity during visceral interoception in weight-restored patients with Anorexia Nervosa. Neuropsychopharmacology **41**(2), 521–528 (2016)
13. Wierenga, C.E., et al.: Hunger does not motivate reward in women remitted from Anorexia Nervosa. Biol Psychiatry **77**(7), 642–652 (2015)

14. Dunn, B.D., et al.: Can you feel the beat? Interoceptive awareness is an interactive function of anxiety- and depression-specific symptom dimensions. Behav Res Ther. **48**(11), 1133–1138 (2010)
15. Pollatos, O., Traut-Mattausch, E., Schandry, R.: Differential effects of anxiety and depression on interoceptive accuracy. Depress Anxiety **26**(2), 167–173 (2009)
16. Sliz, D., Hayley, S.: Major depressive disorder and alterations in insular cortical activity: a review of current functional magnetic imaging research. Front Hum. Neurosci. **6**, 323 (2012)
17. Sprengelmeyer, R., et al.: The insular cortex and the neuroanatomy of major depression. J. Affect. Disord. **133**(1–2), 120–127 (2011)
18. Stephan, K.E., et al.: Allostatic self-efficacy: a metacognitive theory of Dyshomeostasis-induced fatigue and depression. Front. Hum. Neurosci. **10**, 550 (2016)
19. Stratmann, M., et al.: Insular and hippocampal gray matter volume reductions in patients with major depressive disorder. PLoS One **9**(7), e102692 (2014)
20. Wiebking, C., et al.: Interoception in insula subregions as a possible state marker for depression-an exploratory fMRI study investigating healthy, depressed and remitted participants. Front. Behav. Neurosci. **9**, 82 (2015)
21. Naqvi, N.H., Bechara, A.: The hidden island of addiction: the insula. Trends Neurosci. **32** (1), 56–67 (2009)
22. Verdejo-Garcia, A., Clark, L., Dunn, B.D.: The role of interoception in addiction: a critical review. Neurosci. Biobehav. Rev. **36**(8), 1857–1869 (2012)
23. Hughes, K.C., Shin, L.M.: Functional neuroimaging studies of post-traumatic stress disorder. Expert Rev. Neurother. **11**(2), 275–285 (2011)
24. Chen, M.C., et al.: Increased insula coactivation with salience networks in insomnia. Biol. Psychol. **97**, 1–8 (2014)
25. Chatterjee, S.S., Mitra, S.: "I Do Not Exist"—Cotard syndrome in insular cortex atrophy. Biol. Psychiat. **77**(11), e52–e53 (2015)
26. Gorka, S.M., et al.: Insula response to unpredictable and predictable aversiveness in individuals with panic disorder and comorbid depression. Biol. Mood Anxiety Disord. **4**, 9 (2014)
27. Segerdahl, A.R., et al.: The dorsal posterior insula subserves a fundamental role in human pain. Nat. Neurosci. **18**(4), 499–500 (2015)
28. Starr, C.J., et al.: Roles of the insular cortex in the modulation of pain: insights from brain lesions. J. Neurosci. **29**(9), 2684–2694 (2009)
29. Olausson, H., Wessberg, J., Morrison, I., McGlone, F. (eds.): Affective Touch and the Neurophysiology of CT Afferents. Springer, New York (2016). https://doi.org/10.1007/978-1-4939-6418-5
30. Olausson, H., et al.: Unmyelinated tactile afferents signal touch and project to insular cortex. Nat. Neurosci. **5**(9), 900–904 (2002)
31. Crucianelli, L., et al.: Bodily pleasure matters: velocity of touch modulates body ownership during the rubber hand illusion. Front Psychol. **4**, 703 (2013)
32. Crucianelli, L., et al.: The perception of affective touch in Anorexia Nervosa. Psychiatry Res. **239**, 72–78 (2016)
33. Ackerley, R., et al.: Human C-tactile afferents are tuned to the temperature of a skin-stroking caress. J. Neurosci. **34**(8), 2879–2883 (2014)
34. Ogden, R.S., et al.: The effect of pain and the anticipation of pain on temporal perception: a role for attention and arousal. Cogn. Emot. **29**(5), 910–922 (2015)
35. Ogden, R.S., et al.: Stroke me for longer this touch feels too short: the effect of pleasant touch on temporal perception. Conscious Cogn. **36**, 306–313 (2015)
36. Vallbo, A.B., Olausson, H., Wessberg, J.: Unmyelinated afferents constitute a second system coding tactile stimuli of the human hairy skin. J. Neurophysiol. **81**(6), 2753–2763 (1999)

37. Ackerley, R., et al.: Touch perceptions across skin sites: differences between sensitivity, direction discrimination and pleasantness. Front Behav. Neurosci. **8**, 54 (2014)
38. McGlone, F., Wessberg, J., Olausson, H.: Discriminative and affective touch: sensing and feeling. Neuron **82**(4), 737–755 (2014)
39. Wessberg, J., et al.: Receptive field properties of unmyelinated tactile afferents in the human skin. J. Neurophysiol. **89**(3), 1567–1575 (2003)
40. Vallbo, A.B., et al.: Receptive field characteristics of tactile units with myelinated afferents in hairy skin of human subjects. J. Physiol. **483**(Pt 3), 783–795 (1995)
41. Macefield, V.G.: Tactile C fibers. In: Binder, M.D., Hirokawa, N., Windhorst, U. (eds.) Encyclopedia of Neuroscience. Springer, Heidelberg (2009). https://doi.org/10.1007/978-3-540-29678-2
42. Nordin, M.: Low-threshold mechanoreceptive and nociceptive units with unmyelinated (C) fibres in the human supraorbital nerve. J. Physiol. **426**, 229–240 (1990)
43. Liljencrantz, J., Olausson, H.: Tactile C fibers and their contributions to pleasant sensations and to tactile allodynia. Front Behav. Neurosci. **8**, 37 (2014)
44. Di Lernia, D., et al.: Feel the time. Time perception as a function of interoceptive processing. Front. Hum. Neurosci. **12**, 74 (2018)
45. Habig, K., et al.: Low threshold unmyelinated mechanoafferents can modulate pain. BMC Neurol. **17**(1), 184 (2017)
46. Serino, S., et al.: The role of age on multisensory bodily experience: an experimental study with a virtual reality full-body illusion. Cyberpsychol. Behav. Soc. Netw. **21**(5), 304–310 (2018)
47. Zanier, E.R., et al.: Virtual reality for traumatic brain injury. Front. Neurol. **9**, 345 (2018)
48. O'Reilly, J.X., et al.: Dissociable effects of surprise and model update in parietal and anterior cingulate cortex. Proc. Natl. Acad. Sci. USA **110**(38), E3660–E3669 (2013)
49. Rosso, I.M., et al.: Insula and anterior cingulate GABA levels in posttraumatic stress disorder: preliminary findings using magnetic resonance spectroscopy. Depress. Anxiety **31**(2), 115–123 (2014)
50. Di Lernia, D., et al.: Ghosts in the machine interoceptive modeling for chronic pain treatment. Front. Neurosci. **10**, 314 (2016)
51. Riva, G., et al.: Embodied medicine: mens sana in corpore virtuale sano. Front. Hum. Neurosci. **11**, 120 (2017)
52. Riva, G., et al.: Positive and transformative technologies for active ageing. Stud. Health Technol. Inform. **220**, 308–315 (2016)

Learning to Use Tablets After 65:
Auto-regulative Effects of a Training Program

Eleonora Brivio[1,2(✉)], Fabiana Gatti[1], and Carlo Galimberti[1]

[1] Centro Studi e Ricerche di Psicologia della Comunicazione,
Department of Psychology, Università Cattolica del Sacro Cuore,
L.go Gemelli 1, 20123 Milan, Italy
{eleonora.brivio,fabiana.gatti,
carlo.galimberti}@unicatt.it
[2] Clinical and Digital Health Sciences Department,
Augusta University, Augusta, GA, USA
ebrivio@augusta.edu

Abstract. Technology can play a part in the healthy aging process, helping people maintain their social life and remaining cognitively active. Individuals over 65 may have little or no knowledge on how to use technology, therefore they need to learn how to use it before being able to benefit from it. The aim of this paper is to test the efficacy of a digital education program in improving digital self-efficacy, self-esteem, and quality of perception of cognitive skills in older adults. Results show that digital self-efficacy significantly improves, while self-esteem and quality of life increase but not significantly after training. Perception of cognitive skills actually decreased or remain the same after the course.

Keywords: Healthy aging · Digital education · Self-efficacy
Satisfaction with life · Self-esteem · Cognitive abilities · Elderly

1 Introduction

Healthy aging is one of the priorities for many developed countries, as older adults are the fastest growing age bracket. The physical, cognitive, and psychological decline that comes with age can have a negative impact on aging individuals and therefore society: an unhealthy person is unhappy and also costs more in care and assistance. Recent Information and Communication Technologies (ICTs) can be an asset in making life easier and simple during the aging process, as suggested by the Positive Technology paradigm [1]. One of the issue with a wide spread use of technology to promote healthy aging is that many individuals aged 65 and over have little or no knowledge of ICTs: it is paramount therefore to teach older adults how to use technology [2]. In particular, as noted by the DESI country profile [3], in Italy only 43% of the population has basic digital skills (against 55% in Europe) and 63% uses Internet (against 76%), probably due to a large part of the population being 65 years and older. Czaja et al. in 2006 [4] wrote that the digital divide between those aged 65 and the younger generations is caused by external barriers, such as education, finances and physical abilities [5], and

P. Cipresso et al. (Eds.): MindCare 2018, LNICST 253, pp. 50–55, 2018.
https://doi.org/10.1007/978-3-030-01093-5_7

internal factors, such as self-confidence [6], cognitive abilities, and computer anxiety [7, 8]. Training courses are a way of filling this gap in older adults' knowledge.

The aim of this contribution is to examine on an empirical basis if people aged 65 over perceive improvements in their auto-regulative skills (digital self-efficacy, self-esteem), perception of cognitive skills and of satisfaction with life when they take part in a training course designed specifically to teach older adults to use a specific technology (tablet).

1.1 Technology and the Older Adult

It is important for older adults to learn how to use technology because technology-based services and interactions are increasingly part of daily life and are essential to a heathy aging process. Auto-regulative skills and cognitive abilities come into play into this learning process.

Many older adults have little or no intention to learn, adopt, and use new technological devices, mostly because they have negative attitudes towards ICTs and low levels of Self-Efficacy [9]. Self-Efficacy is the belief a person has in his or her ability and skills to perform a task [10]. A low ICT-specific Self-Efficacy is therefore to be taken into account when older adults learn how to use technology. Perceived cognitive abilities (belief about memory, concentration, etc.) also may contribute to the belief of efficacy [11].

Similarly, Self Esteem is a (positive or negative) feeling of self-worth and is strongly connected to the experiences one has [12]: having positive experiences and achieving goals improve Self-Esteem. In particular, engaging in an experience to learn technology successfully can increase confidence and self-esteem in older adults [13]. Another overall evaluation of a person's experience over the course of his or her life is Life Satisfaction [14].

If the ICT learning experience can improve older adults' Digital Self Efficacy, their perception of cognitive skills, Self-Esteem, and overall Life Satisfaction may also increase.

1.2 Research Questions

The research had the following hypotheses:

H_1: Digital Self-Efficacy scores increase after the course in comparison to the baseline.

H_2: Life Satisfaction and Self Esteem levels improve after training in comparison to the baseline.

H_3: Perception of Cognitive Skills is higher at the end of the training in comparison to the beginning of the course.

2 Methodology

A longitudinal design was used for this study: participants were assessed before starting the training course and after the last session of the course. Total time between measurements was 12 weeks. Paired Sample T-Tests were used to assess differences between baseline and after course scores.

2.1 The Training Course

A total of 50 participants was divided into four groups and took part to the training. The course consisted of ten two-hour lessons where a group of 10–12 participants was trained in the use of tablets by a professional trainer and assisted by two tutors. Each class included a theory based introduction of the topic and the specific lexicon for the class, followed by practical exercise on the tablet. The course lasted 10 weeks, with one class help per week. The theoretical bases for the training are explained in detail elsewhere [15].

2.2 Measurements

The measures used in this study were the following. The research used the Italian validated version of each measure.

Digital Self Efficacy Questionnaire: A 23-item questionnaire with a 5-point likert scale, created to test self-efficacy with a tablet [16]. The questionnaire has two dimensions: a general digital self-efficacy scale, measuring the confidence people have with the basic functioning of the tablet (e.g. the operating system, writing, etc.), and an app-specific scale, measuring the confidence with using app to carry out specific tasks.

Life Satisfaction Index – Version A (LSIA-11): the LSIA-11 is a 11 item measure of perception of one's satisfaction with life. It has three subscales: Mood Tone, Zest for Life, and Congruence between desired and achieved goals [17].

Rosenberg's Self Esteem Questionnaire: The Italian version of this measure is a 10 item global score scale that assesses a person's self-esteem [18]. It's unidimensional.

Cognitive Failure Questionnaire: This instrument assesses an individual's perception of errors in the area of memory (general and memory of names), concentration, distractibility, and personal intelligence [19]. It comprises of 25 items on a 5 point Likert scale.

2.3 Sample

The sample of this study is composed of 50 people aged 65 and over, recruited through a Lifelong Learning center in Milan, Italy.

Thirty-five participants (74.5%) were women. Mean age for the sample is 70.68 year old. The sample has a high level education, with 57.4% (n = 27) of the participants having a high school diploma and another 23.4% (n = 11) having a university degree.

Twenty-eight participants (60%) had already attended a training course for technology (computer or tablet) at the time of the study.

3 Results

Table 1 shows the results for the Paired Sample T-Test in the two dimensions of Digital Self-Efficacy: changes in mean were highly significant, with measurements after the course having higher scores than baseline.

Table 1. Results for the digital self efficacy paired sample T-test

	m_{t1}	sd_{t1}	m_{t2}	sd_{t2}	T	df	Sig.
General digital self efficacy	0.98	0.66	2.36	0.71	−13.53	38	.001
App specific self efficacy	1.05	0.67	2.43	0.64	−12.53	38	.001

Paired Sample T Test for the Rosenberg Self-Esteem indicated no significant change (t(38) = −.043, p = .966). Average score at baseline was m = 23.77, ds = 2.66, while at the end of the course it was m = 23.80, ds = 3.00, showing a slight upward trend.

Results for the dimensions of Satisfaction with life are in Table 2. The analysis did not reveal any significant changes in mean scores, even though the Zest for Life subscale presented a trend toward significance and the participants scored slightly higher after the course.

Table 2. Results for the LSIA-11 paired sample T-test

	m_{t1}	sd_{t1}	m_{t2}	sd_{t2}	T	df	Sig.
Mood tone	.80	.41	.85	.50	−.569	38	.572
Zest for life	.75	.36	.86	.32	−1.81	38	.077
Congruence	1.43	.57	1.48	.57	−.506	38	.616

The mean comparison for the Cognitive Failure Questionnaire (Table 3) pointed out to significant difference between before and after the course scores in two dimensions: Memory and Concentration. In both cases, average scores decreased significantly in T_2.

Table 3. Results for the cognitive failure questionnaire paired sample T-test

	m_{t1}	sd_{t1}	m_{t2}	sd_{t2}	T	df	Sig.
Memory	1.42	.59	1.19	.52	3.876	38	.001
Memory for names	1.67	.81	1.68	.94	−.119	38	.898
Concentration	1.92	.56	1.43	.65	7.681	38	.001
Distractibility	1.10	.57	1.08	.64	.332	38	.742
Personal intelligence	1.32	.67	1.33	.72	−.114	37	.906

4   Discussion and Conclusion

The hypotheses were only partially supported by the data.

In particular, Digital Self Efficacy improved significantly after the course, suggesting that training is viable path to make older adult more familiar and confident with a technological device. The training program seems to help participants to be more confident in handling the tablet: more in the app-specific Self Efficacy than general Digital Self Efficacy. The design of the IOS may explain the differences in General Digital Self Efficacy and App-Specific Self Efficacy: the operating system interface seems not to be linear, and thus generate difficulties in handling the tablet in its basic functions, while apps work linearly and thus are easier to handle for older adults.

Other auto-regulative skills did not show significant increase with the training, even though the upward trend of the scores suggest that the training may have more effect if it lasted longer and had a more intense schedule. Both Satisfaction with Life and Self-Esteem are general constructs that are built in time. The time of the training and actual use of the tablet was limited: only few participants had a tablet at home and could practice and use it in the context of their own lives. Therefore, both time between measurements and lack of actual use in context may have contributed to non-significant results in Self-Esteem and Satisfaction with Life. It is also worth noting that starting average scores for this sample are high. Future studies should also use more domain-specific measures and try to gauge the effects of the training with a follow up measurement one month or more after the training is over.

Rising difficulty in the course appears to make people less confident in their memory and concentration skills, probably because of the number of information needed to handle the tablet's more complex functions: it is necessary to calibrate better the courses, or to collect data not at the end of the class (when the participant's energy is depleted), but maybe half a day later after the end of the class and of the course.

One of the limitations of the study is the sample, which is limited to fifty people, who were all recruited from the same Learning Center. The participants were all already involved in learning: in the future, research should also focus on investigating the power of technology not just to close the generational divide but to promote social inclusion of other underserved, fragile populations (e.g. low income, low levels of education) who are not already involved in learning contexts: the training was proved to be effective in teaching older adults how to use tablets, and therefore can be used with different and larger populations.

Acknowledgments. This work is supported by the D3.2 2014 Progetti di Interesse d'Ateneo scheme, Università Cattolica del Sacro Cuore, Milan, Italy.

References

1. Riva, G., Banos, R.M., Botella, C., Wienderhold, B.K., Gaggioli, A.: Positive techology: using interactive technologies to promote positive functioning. Cyberpsychol. Behav. Soc. Netw. **15**, 69–77 (2012)
2. Kim, Y.S.: Reviewing and critiquing computer leaning and usage among older adults. Educ. Gerontol. **34**, 709–735 (2008)
3. Digital Economy and Society Index 2016 (DESI): Italy Country Profile. https://ec.europa.eu/digital-single-market/en/scoreboard/italy
4. Cazaja, S., et al.: Factors predicting the use of technology: finding from the Center for Research and Education and Aging and Technology Enhancement (CREATE). Psychol. Aging **21**, 333–352 (2006)
5. Pew Internet & American life Project: Generation online in 2009. http://www.pewinternet.org/2009/01/28/generations-online-in-2009/
6. Purdie, N., Boulton-Lewis, G.: The learning needs of older adults. Educ. Gerontol. **29**, 129–149 (2003)
7. Broady, T., Chan, A., Caputi, P.: Comparison of older and younger adults' attitudes towards and abilities with computers: implication for training and learning. Br. J. Educ. Technol. **41**, 473–485 (2010)
8. Mitzner, T., et al.: Older adults' training preferences for learning to use technology. In: Proceedings of the Human Factors and Ergonomics Society 52nd Annual Meeting, vol. 52, no. 26, pp. 2047–2051 (2008)
9. González, A., Ramírez, M.P., Viadel, V.: Attitudes of the elderly toward information and communications technologies. Educ. Gerontol. **38**, 585–594 (2012)
10. Bandura, A.: Self-efficacy: the exercise of control. Freeman, New York (1997)
11. Bandura, A.: Perceived self-efficacy in cognitive development and functioning. Educ. Psychol. **28**, 117–148 (1993)
12. Baumeister, R.F., Smart, L., Boden, J.: Relation of threatened egotism to violence and aggression: the dark side of self-esteem. Psychol. Rev. **103**, 5–33 (1996)
13. Gatto, S.L., Tak, S.H.: Computer, internet, and e-mail use among older adults. Educ. Gerontol. **34**, 800–811 (2008)
14. Diener, E., Emmons, R.A., Larsen, R.J., Griffin, S.: The satisfaction with life scale. J. Pers. Asses. **49**, 71–75 (1985)
15. Gatti, F., Brivio, E., Galimberti, C.: "The Future Is Ours Too": a training process to enable the learning perception and increase self-efficacy in the use of tablet in the elderly. Educ. Gerontol. **43**, 209–224 (2017)
16. Brivio, E., Serino, S., Galimberti, C., Riva, G.: Efficacy of a digital education program in life satisfaction and digital self efficacy in older adults: a mixed method study. Ann. Rev. Cyber. Ther. Telemed. **14**, 45–50 (2016)
17. Franchignoni, F., Tesio, L., Ottonello, M., Benevolo, E.: Life satisfaction index: Italian version and validation of a short form. Am. J. Phys. Med. Rehabil. **78**, 509–515 (1999)
18. Prezza, M., Trombaccia, F.R., Armento, L.: La Scala dell'Autostima di Rosenberg: Traduzione e Validazione Italiana. B. Psicol. Appl. **223**, 35–44 (1997)
19. Stratta, P., Rinaldi, O., Daneluzzo, E., Rossi, A.: Utilizzo della Versione Italiana del Cognitive Failure Questionnaire (CFQ) in un Campione di Studenti: Uno Studio di Validazione. Riv. Psichiatr. **41**, 260–265 (2006)

Learning into the Wild: A Protocol for the Use of 360° Video for Foreign Language Learning

Claudia Repetto[1]([✉]), Serena Germagnoli[1], Stefano Triberti[1], and Giuseppe Riva[1,2]

[1] Department of Psychology, Catholic University of Sacred Heart,
L.go Gemelli 1, Milan, Italy
{claudia.repetto, stefano.triberti,
giuseppe.riva}@unicatt.it,
serena.germagnoli@gmail.com
[2] Applied Technology for Neuropsychology Laboratory,
IRCCS Istituto Auxologico Italiano, Via Magnasco 2, Milan, Italy

Abstract. Learning a second language could be a boring task if accomplished by repeating bilingual words lists. Laboratory research demonstrated that second language learning is more efficient if the material is enriched by pictures or gestures during the encoding phase. Here we want to test the impact of 360° videos on foreign language learning. The 360° videos are spherical videos that allow a lifelike exploration of the environment, if experienced immersively (namely, by means of a Head Mounted Display). The protocol includes ten 360° videos representing natural landscapes, sport performances and adventures; each video has been enriched with a narrative that guides the subject's attention towards the relevant elements named in English (the second language). The goals are twofold: first, we want to investigate whether the videos fruition is able to promote language learning; second, we want to verify the acceptability and perceived utility of this technology by potential users.

Keywords: Virtual Reality · 360° video · Second language learning Embodied Cognition

1 Theoretical Background

Traditional cognitive models of human mind considered our brain as a computer manipulating abstract symbols that follow predefined formal rules [1, 2]. According to this view, superior mental processes, such as problem solving, comprehension, recall of memories, operate on representations detached from sensory-motor experiences. An alternative and increasingly more influential view is the Embodied Cognition approach, which encompasses slightly different theoretical accounts, though associated by a fundamental core position: according to this perspective, the Cartesian dichotomy between mind and body is deemed incorrect, since mental operations are strictly related to, and dependent from, our bodies [3, 4]. Embodied theories of cognition extended the boundaries of anatomical structures to which traditionally a specific function was assigned: the mind is no longer confined to the brain but also includes other body parts,

P. Cipresso et al. (Eds.): MindCare 2018, LNICST 253, pp. 56–63, 2018.
https://doi.org/10.1007/978-3-030-01093-5_8

such as hands, legs, eyes. Moreover, within the brain, the separation between primary areas, recruited for basic sensory and motor processing, and the associative areas, in which more complex processes take place, is not strictly defined anymore: actually, the distinction between low and high level processes drops down in favor of a more integrated model. This new model proposes an interplay that allows the recruitment of primary areas even during "superior" cognitive processes: therefore, according to this account, the neural structures involved in sensory, perceptual or motor areas are also active when we construct concepts, make inferences, recall memories and use language. Although the perceptual and sensory system and their influence on cognitive processing have been investigated [5–7], without a doubt the motor system assumed a very special role in this line of research. The importance of the motor system is well recognizable in Wilson's words [8], *"Cognition is for action. The function of the mind is to guide action, and cognitive mechanisms such as perception and memory must be understood in terms of their ultimate contribution to situation-appropriate behaviour"* (p. 626). Of note, the link between the motor and the cognitive systems is bidirectional: if cognition is for action it is also suggested that action influences cognition [9].

In this study we will focus on the effects of action towards language processing. The idea that language and motor system are not independent, nor free from reciprocal influences is not that recent: the Lieberman's Motor Theory of Speech Perception [10, 11] is one of the first theoretical proposals in this direction. In the last decades, however, a huge amount of experimental proofs demonstrated the crosstalk between the two systems. At a behavioral level, performing an action while processing language has specific consequences on the latter. For example, in the classical Action- sentence Compatibility Effect (ACE) paradigm [12], participants are required to make sensibility judgments on sentences that describe actions towards the body ("John opens the drawer") or away from the body ("John closes the drawer"). Crucially, the response is provided by making an arm movement either away or towards one's body; the effect is underlined by faster reaction times in providing the response when the action performed by the participant matches that described in the sentence.

Another way to use action in connection with language is through object manipulation. It has been demonstrated that children, who act out a just read sentence by means of toys representing the sentence components, perform better on a comprehension task compared to other children that only read the sentence [13–15]. It has been suggested that the manipulation task forces the child to connect words to particular objects and syntactic relations to actions, resulting in better comprehension of the sentence [16].

An important line of research in the investigation of the effects of action on language is dedicated to the study of second language learning (L2). In the next paragraph the topic will be explored by introducing the concept of enrichment and its beneficial effects on learning.

2 Enrichment in Foreign Language Learning

Studying a foreign language could be a boring task if the learner tries to memorizes bilingual words lists. However, the task could become more engaging and the performance more efficient if the words are enriched by other stimuli. Empirical studies have shown that multisensory enrichment promotes verbal learning [17]. The reason why enrichment enhances memory performance is accounted for by two influential cognitive theories: the Dual Code Theory [18] and the Level of Processing Theory [19]. According to the Dual Code Theory, the combination of visual and verbal information during the encoding phase yields better memory performance. If words are recalled, one of the two codes (either visual or verbal) is available. The Level of Processing Framework (LOP) predicts that memory outcome depends on the "degree of depth" achieved during information encoding. If verbal information (in this case, a word) is encoded in a shallow way (i.e., at the phonological level by only hearing it), the recall of that word will be less efficient than if it were processed deeply, at the semantic level. In this respect, enriching a word, either by adding sensorimotor information to it or by processing it semantically, can enhance its depth of processing, consequently making it more resistant to decay.

Enrichment can be accomplished in different ways: a flash card representing the word's semantics can accompany the novel word during learning. Additionally, the motor system can be recruited to enrich the written word. This is done by performing an action or a gesture connected to the word [20, 21]. Literature in action memory investigates the role of a self-performed action (SPT) in the recall of action sentences (usually short phrases composed of an action verb plus an object) compared to either observing the experimenter performing the action (EPT) or verbal encoding alone (VE). In experiments, participants learning in the SPT condition show better memory performance compared to those in the EPT and VE condition [22]. This indicates that the motor component has a greater impact on retention if the action or gesture is self-performed than if the action is only observed. The superiority of the SPT is often referred to as the "enactment effect" (EE) [23].

A parallel line of research investigates the enactment effect on word learning in a second language (L2). Studies in this field target the impact of different kinds of gestures in word retention. These studies compare the effect of gestures on memory for words to the effect of other enriching methods (e.g., with pictures). Tellier [24] trained 20 French pre-schoolers with eight English words associated with self-performed gestures and with pictures. Memory performance was better for words encoded with gestures than for those encoded with pictures. In a combined fMRI and behavioral study, Macedonia et al. [25] explored the impact of iconic versus meaningless gestures on L2 words in a sample of young adults. This experiment was designed to determine whether the memory enhancement comes from the motor trace created by the action/gesture used in the word's representation or from the gestures' semantics. If the benefit derives from the gestures' semantics, then words encoded with iconic gestures should be remembered better than those encoded with a meaningless gesture. On the other hand, if the motor component per se would impact memory, the two encoding conditions should yield the same results in memory performance. Behavioral data indicated that better performance relies on the gestural semantics. This finding was confirmed in a study by Mayer et al. [26], where German subjects learned new words under different enrichment conditions: performing an iconic gesture, seeing an associated picture, copying the outline of the picture with the index finger, or no enrichment. After five days of training, participants recalled words encoded with iconic gestures better compared to words encoded in all the other experimental conditions.

In the present protocol we want to test the effect of another type of enrichment, that is the naturalistic exploration of a virtual environment. Virtual Reality is the ideal medium where a multisensory environment can be implemented. It allows the user to feel a high sense of presence within the environment thanks to its tridimensional graphics and, especially, the opportunities of exploration [27]. Previous studies already employed Virtual Reality in the field of second language acquisition [28]. Some decades ago, Rose and Billinghurst [29] set up a fully immersive VR application to teach Japanese prepositions. In their approach, learners were trained with a three-step protocol: first, they freely explored the virtual environment, wherein the objects could be touched in order to hear their name and color from a digitalized voice; second, they watched animation sequences and used vocal commands; third, the played a virtual game where they had to assemble stacks of blocks matching samples shapes presented. More recently, Amoia and collaborators [30] presented I-FLEG a serious game designed to interactively learn French as second language. The game is exploited within Second Life environment (http://secondlife.com/). Connecting to the Allegro Island the user enters a 3D environment populated by different houses, each of whom is a different learning unit. Exploring the houses, the learner can train lexical domains or grammar, and the content varies depending on the individual's proficiency. This game is highly sophisticated as it offers targeted feedbacks and modular learning units, but is not immersive, since it is not designed to be used with a HMD.

In this study we aim to employ enriched 360° videos displayed on the smartphone and experienced immersively by means of a cardboard, to improve second language learning in high school students.

3 Experimental Protocol

3.1 Material

Ten 360° videos have been selected, among those available on the web, with the purpose of catching the adolescents' attention. 360° videos are spherical videos recorded by means of special camera with omnidirectional lenses. During the playback, a user, after having worn a cardboard, can control the viewing direction by means of the head movement in a very realistic way (looking up one can see the sky/roof, looking down one can see the floor/ground, and if one wants to see what happens on the left/right, it is sufficient to turn the head accordingly, as in the real life situations). Of note, within 360° videos it is not possible to select the direction of the navigation, nor to interact with the elements of the environment.

Selected videos represent natural landscapes, sport performances, adventures and interior environments.

Each video was carefully inspected to identify the relevant elements included and the actions performed by the characters. Scenes were extracted that represented elements whose label are both at high and low frequency in the second language (Mean frequency = 168.87; sta. dev. = 316.48, according to COLFIS, Corpus e Lessico di Frequenza dell'Italiano Scritto [31]). High frequency words are supposed to be already known by the students, but still they are useful to make the user feel confident with the task and to improve his/her self-efficacy. After having selected the scenes, objects and actions displayed within them were listed and become the target words to be learned in the second language (namely English, for the Italian native speakers). Afterwards, a narrative was created that connected them into a coherent story. The narrative has the purpose to guide the user's attention and focus it towards the target elements named. An English mother tongue woman audio recorded the narratives, and the audio file was added to the video in the post-production phase, synchronizing the speech to the images displayed. Duration ranges from 30 s to 1 min and 30 s. In the end, the user playing the video can experience the environment as if (s)he was in a foreign country with a native speaker talking to him/her and illustrating the environment in which both are navigating.

3.2   Procedure

This study is targeted to high school students studying English as second language.

The protocol includes two sessions in the classroom during regular lessons, with one month of delay in the between. An outline of the research protocol is represented in Fig. 1.

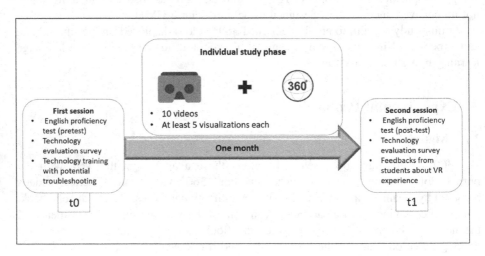

Fig. 1. The protocol of the research

First Session (T0) → During this session a series of pretests will be conducted. First, the baseline English knowledge will be assessed by presenting the students with the lists of item trained within the videos and asking them to translate from Italian into

Table 1. Items of the technology evaluation survey used during the first session.

1. I think that Virtual Reality will help me to improve my skills
2. I think that Virtual Reality-based training will improve my English proficiency
3. I think that Virtual Reality is useful
4. I think that learning to use Virtual Reality will be easy for me
5. I think it will be easy for me becoming a Virtual Reality expert
6. I think that Virtual Reality is easy to use
7. I'm going to use Virtual Reality regularly

English the words they know. Second, the attitude of the students towards the technology employed will be evaluated. To this purpose a brief survey will be administered, in which one has to claim the degree of agreement with the sentences presented. According to the Technology Acceptance Model [32], sentences cover two main topics: perceived ease of use and perceived utility. The complete list of sentences is reported in Table 1.

The session ends with a training illustrating the use of the cardboard, the videos' downloading and fruition by means of commercial Applications, and a potential troubleshooting phase to fix issues arisen with the personal mobile device.

Individual study → it lasts about 1 month, in which the students are requested to watch the videos individually, at home. A detailed program of visualization is provided, that combines the need to maximize the learning opportunities and the need to prevent side effects (each video should be watched at least five times, no more than 5 min of training are recommended, at least 2 h should pass between two consecutive trainings).

Second Session (T1) → During this session a series of post-tests will be conducted. First, memory performance for the trained words will be assessed: the students will undergo the same bilingual translation task administered in the First Session. Second, students will compile the technology evaluation survey claiming their opinion about the virtual experience and reporting potential side effects encountered. Free comments and suggestions will be collected for further tuning of the technologies or the protocol. Also, students will be asked to report, as an approximate percentage, how much of the expected program of visualization they think to have actually completed: this would allow to compare actual use with users' previous expectations and evaluations, according to the Technology Acceptance Model [32]. Third, students will be asked to evaluate the sense of presence they felt within each 360° video experience. It should be taken into account that 360° videos do not allow interaction except for visually exploring the environment, and interaction (or the perceived possibility for it) is considered one of the main factors impacting on sense of presence [27]. Anyway, the sense of presence is still considered one of the main aspects to monitor in order to evaluate the efficacy of immersive technologies [27]. In order to provide a "presence score" which would make available for researcher to compare single videos' effectiveness, students will be familiarized with the concept of presence by means of a short debriefing; then, they will be asked to rate the level of presence they experienced in each 360° video, as previously done in the literature [33].

4 Expected Results

This protocol will allow us to collect several information about the potential use of the 360° video for second language learning. First, by comparing the students' performance in the pre and post sessions we can test the efficacy of the protocol in terms of new words learned: we expect a significant improvement of the vocabulary after the training. More, we are interested in investigating the impact of the personal attitudes towards technology on the learning process: we expect that students having positive expectations about the ease of use and the utility of the videos will learn more efficiently, indicating that the technology is not "preferable" per se, but strongly interacts with motivation and beliefs. However, it is possible that the post sessions evaluations of the technology are better predictors of the learning performance, indicating that, despite the initial skepticism about the potential usefulness and ease of use, a positive experience is able to promote an efficient learning. Finally, by analyzing presence rates, it will be possible to identify a set of videos more likely to constitute an effective resource for second language learning.

Acknowledgments. This work was partially supported by Fondazione Cassa di Risparmio di Alessandria.

References

1. Fodor, J.A.: The Modularity of Mind. MIT press, Cambridge (1983)
2. Fodor, J.A.: The Language of Thought. Harvard University Press, Cambridge (1975)
3. Barsalou, L.W.: Grounded cognition. Annu. Rev. Psychol. **59**, 617–645 (2008)
4. Shapiro, L.A.: Embodied Cognition. Routledge, Abingdon (2011)
5. Martin, A., Haxby, J.V., Lalonde, F.M., Wiggs, C.L., Ungerleider, L.G.: Discrete cortical regions associated with knowledge of color and knowledge of action. Science (80-) **270**, 102–105 (1995)
6. Goldberg, R.F., Perfetti, C.A., Schneider, W.: Perceptual knowledge retrieval activates sensory brain regions. J. Neurosci. **26**, 4917–4921 (2006)
7. Thompson-Schill, S.L.: Neuroimaging studies of semantic memory: inferring 'how' from 'where'. Neuropsychologia **41**, 280–292 (2003)
8. Wilson, M.: Six views of embodied cognition. Psychon. Bull. Rev. **9**, 625–636 (2002)
9. Glenberg, A.M.: What memory is for. Behav. Brain Sci. **20**, 1–55 (1997)
10. Galantucci, B., Fowler, C.A., Turvey, M.T.: The motor theory of speech perception reviewed. Psychon. Bull. Rev. **13**, 361–377 (2006)
11. Liberman, A.M., Mattingly, I.G.: The motor theory of speech perception. Cognition **21**, 1–36 (1985)
12. Glenberg, A.M., Kaschak, M.P.: Grounding language in action. Psychon. Bull. Rev. **9**, 558–565 (2002)
13. Glenberg, A.M., Gutierrez, T., Levin, J.R., Japuntich, S., Kaschak, M.P.: Activity and imagined activity can enhance young children's reading comprehension. J. Educ. Psychol. **96**, 424–436 (2004)
14. Glenberg, A.M., Brown, M., Levin, J.R.: Enhancing comprehension in small reading groups using a manipulation strategy. Contemp. Educ. Psychol. **32**, 389–399 (2007)

15. Marley, S.C., Levin, J.R., Glenberg, A.M.: Improving Native American children's listening comprehension through concrete representations. Contemp. Educ. Psychol. **32**, 537–550 (2007)
16. Glenberg, A.M., Goldberg, A.B., Zhu, X.: Improving early reading comprehension using embodied CAI. Instr. Sci. **39**, 27–39 (2011)
17. Shams, L., Seitz, A.R.: Benefits of multisensory learning. Trends Cogn. Sci. **12**, 411–417 (2008)
18. Paivio, A., Csapo, K.: Concrete image and verbal memory codes. J. Exp. Psychol. **80**, 279 (1969)
19. Craik, F.I.M., Tulving, E.: Depth of processing and the retention of words in episodic memory. J. Exp. Psychol. Gen. **104**, 268–294 (1975)
20. Macedonia, M., von Kriegstein, K.: Gestures enhance foreign language learning. Biolinguistics **6**, 393–416 (2012)
21. Zimmer, H.D., et al.: Memory for Action: A Distinct for of Episodic Memory?. Oxford University Press, Oxford (2001)
22. Nilsson, L.G.: Remembering actions and words. In: Tulving, E., Craik, F.I.M. (eds.) The Oxford Handbook of Memory, pp. 137–148. Oxford University Press (2000)
23. Engelkamp, J.: Memory for Actions. Psychology Press/Taylor & Francis, Hove/Abingdon (1998)
24. Tellier, M.: The effect of gestures on second language memorisation by young children. Gesture **8**, 219–235 (2008)
25. Macedonia, M., Knösche, T.R.: Body in mind: how gestures empower foreign language learning. Mind Brain Educ. **5**, 196–211 (2011)
26. Mayer, K.M., Yildiz, I.B., Macedonia, M., Von Kriegstein, K.: Visual and motor cortices differentially support the translation of foreign language words. Curr. Biol. **25**, 530–535 (2015)
27. Triberti, S., Riva, G.: Being present in action: a theoretical model about the 'interlocking' between intentions and environmental affordances. Front. Psychol. **6**, 2052 (2016)
28. Schwienhorst, K.: The state of VR: a meta-analysis of virtual reality tools in second language acquisition. Comput. Assist. Lang. Learn. **15**, 221–239 (2002)
29. Rose, H., Billinghurst, M.: Zengo Sayu: an immersive educational environment for learning Japanese (1995)
30. Amoia, M., et al.: A serious game for second language acquisition in a virtual environment. J. Syst. Cybern. Inform. **10**, 24–34 (2012)
31. Bertinetto, P., et al.: Corpus e Lessico di Frequenza dell'Italiano Scritto (CoLFIS) (2005). http://linguistica.sns.it/CoLFIS/Home.htm
32. Davis, F.D.: Perceived usefulness, perceived ease of use and user acceptance information technology. MIS Q. **13**, 319–339 (1989)
33. IJsselsteijn, W., de Riddera, H., Hamberga, R., Bouwhuisa, D., Freeman, J.: Perceived depth and the feeling of presence in 3DTV. Displays **18**, 207–214 (1998)

The Technology-Enhanced Ability Continuum-of-Care Home Program for People with Cognitive Disorders: Concept Design and Scenario of Use

Olivia Realdon[1(✉)], Federica Rossetto[2], Marco Nalin[3], Ilaria Baroni[3],
Maria Romano[3], Felice Catania[4], David Frontini[4],
Sergio Mancastroppa[4], Margherita Alberoni[2], Valentino Zurloni[1],
Raffaello Nemni[2,5], Fabrizia Mantovani[1],
Francesca Baglio[2], and The Ability Consortium

[1] Università degli Studi di Milano-Bicocca,
P.zza Ateneo Nuovo, 1, 20126 Milan, Italy
{olivia.realdon,valentino.zurloni,
fabrizia.mantovani}@unimib.it
[2] IRCCS Fondazione don Carlo Gnocchi, via Capecelatro, 66, Milan, Italy
{frossetto,malberoni,rnemni,fbaglio}@dongnocchi.it
[3] Telbios S.r.l, Research & Development, via Olgettina, 60, 20132 Milan, Italy
{marco.nalin,ilaria.baroni,maria.romano}@telbios.com
[4] Astir S.r.l, IT Development, via Giovanni Battista Pirelli, 30,
20124 Milan, Italy
{felice.catania,david.frontini,
sergio.mancastroppa}@astir.com
[5] Department of Pathophysiology and Transplantation,
Università degli Studi di Milano, via Francesco Sforza 35, 20122 Milan, Italy

Abstract. Alzheimer's disease (AD) has been identified as one of the 25 top causes of years lived with disability. Currently, no pharmacological treatment can prevent, slow down, or stop the course of this disease. From the clinical and health management perspectives, Mild Cognitive Impairment – a condition representing a risk factor for the development of dementia - and early stages of AD are the most interesting conditions for interventions aimed at delaying further decline. Telemonitoring and telerehabilitation home-based services have been advocated to provide manifold benefits for people with cognitive disorders. In this paper, we will describe the concept vision enlightening Ability, a technology-enhanced continuity-of-care home program for people with cognitive disorders. After describing the platform architecture, we will present a use case showing how it benefits people with cognitive disorders and both formal and informal caregivers by generating intertwining support in the process of care, enhancing well-being, health conditions, and inclusion.

Keywords: Telerehabilitation · Cognitive disorders · Alzheimer's disease
Dementia · Cognitive rehabilitation

© ICST Institute for Computer Sciences, Social Informatics and Telecommunications Engineering 2018
P. Cipresso et al. (Eds.): MindCare 2018, LNICST 253, pp. 64–73, 2018.
https://doi.org/10.1007/978-3-030-01093-5_9

1 Introduction

Currently, about one-eighth of life expectancy worldwide is associated with disability [1]. An epidemiological shift was detected between 1990 and 2013, showing increasing numbers for non-communicable diseases and, at the same time, decreasing rates for communicable disorders. Among non-communicable disorders, Alzheimer's disease (AD) has been identified among the 25 top causes of years lived with disability [2].

AD is the most common form of dementia, being a progressive neurodegenerative condition accounting for up to 60% of all dementia cases [3]. From the clinical and health management point of view, Mild Cognitive Impairment (MCI) – a condition representing a risk factor for the development of dementia - and early stages of AD are the most interesting target for interventions aimed at preventing or delaying further decline [4]. So far, no pharmacological therapy is available to prevent the potential conversion from an MCI to an AD condition, or to affect the course of AD.

Nevertheless, different types of non-pharmacological interventions have been conceived to meet this challenge and an increasing body of results shows that cognitive functions of people with mild to moderate dementia benefit from cognitive stimulation programs, over and above any medication effects [5]. However, to consolidate this evidence, the adoption of robust experimental designs and validated and reliable measures of efficacy on both cognitive and non-cognitive (i.e., Quality of Life; QoL) outcomes is still crucial [6]. Furthermore, among non-pharmacological interventions, using technology to provide a range of home-based services has currently gained importance [7]. Several benefits of these long-distance monitoring and rehabilitation services have been highlighted. For instance, these services provide equitable access to local sanitary systems for individuals who are geographically remote and/or with physical disabilities [8], remote therapeutic interventions and monitoring of progress, lower costs, and support of the person with dementia-caregiver dyads at home [9, 10]. Indeed, computer-based interventions are often cited in many literature reviews on cognitive interventions, [5, 11, 12] because of the opportunities they provide in terms of fine-grained adjustments and individual tailoring of intensity and duration of cognitive rehabilitation/stimulation programs. Nonetheless, the lack of familiarity of older adults with technologies and computers is often raised as a potential obstacle for their adoption [13].

Within this scenario, the technology-enhanced Ability continuity-of-care home program for people with cognitive disorders has recently been devised within the Ability Project, funded within the Smart Cities and Communities Funding Program (MIUR-POR LOMBARDY; AXIS 1; POR FESR 2007–2013). The Ability project Consortium included industries and SMEs, Research institutions, and PAs, which received an overall funding of 4,08 MI euros.

In this paper we will first focus on the architecture of the platform, designed and developed to enable the continuity-of-care Ability program. We will then present a use case highlighting how it benefits both people with cognitive disorders and formal and informal caregivers by the generation of continuous and intertwining support in the process of care.

2   The Technology-Enhanced Ability Continuity-of-Care Home Program for People with Cognitive Disorders: Platform Architecture and Use Scenario

The technology-enhanced Ability continuity-of-care home program targeted the design, development and validation of a smart care environment. The aim of such program was to foster inclusion, well-being, and health conditions of people with cognitive disorders, providing continuous support to their caregivers at the same time.

The vision of the Ability program was to develop and test a Personal Smart Care Community enabling innovative trajectories for dementia care. Such Community puts the patient at the core of an intertwining treatment and support from both formal (e.g. physicians) and informal (e.g. near relatives) caregivers while moving from hospital-based to home-based care.

To reach this aim, the designed and developed Ability platform represents a tool to monitor vital parameters remotely, and to deliver motor and cognitive rehabilitation activities.

The system of the Ability platform is based on the Telbios Connect, a telemonitoring platform for chronic patients already existing prior to the design and development of the Ability continuity-of-care program. The architecture of the Telbios Connect platform, with the Ability vertical application integrated in it, is shown in Fig. 1.

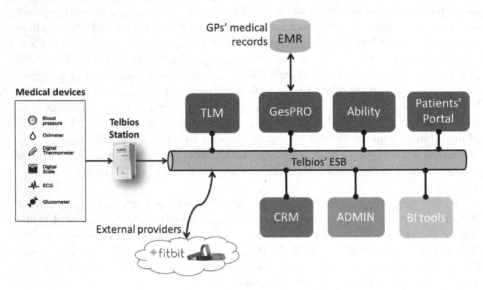

Fig. 1. The architecture of the Telbios Connect platform with the Ability vertical application integrated.

The Telbios Connect platform is centered on an Enterprise Service Bus (ESB) that connects all proprietary and third party applications. Besides administrative (ADMIN) and Business Intelligence Tools (BI Tools), the platform provides a Customer

Relationship Management (CRM) tool, which the Telbios Service Center uses to manage users in the different services. The ESB also allows the integration and exchange of data with external services (e.g., Fitbit APIs) or hardware, such as the Telbios Station, a residential gateway that connects Bluetooth self-monitoring devices.

On top of this core infrastructure, vertical applications can be developed in order to benefit from the exchange of information. Among these, for example, the GesPRO allows General Practitioners (GPs) to manage chronic patients, prescribing yearly care plans and monitoring their statuses. The telemonitoring application (TLM) allows the collection of vital parameters such as weight, heart rate, ECGs, SpO2, blood pressure and blood glucose, based on a Telemonitoring Plan (TP) defined by a clinician. Moreover, the platform can analyze the data from vital parameters in real time and activate specific protocols of escalation on nurses or physicians, depending on the severity of the identified condition of the patient.

During the design and development of the Ability continuity-of-care home program, the platform was extended to include also: (a) data coming from commercial actigraphy devices (i.e., the Fitbit tracker), hosting motor activity and sleep behavior data; (b) motor and cognitive rehabilitation contents, developed ad-hoc for the program or hosted on third party platforms, and a defined interface for results exchange.

Using Telbios Connect as a starting point, the Ability application was then built around the concept of Individual Rehabilitation Plan (IRP). In the Ability continuity-of-care program, the IRP includes cognitive rehabilitation activities (a library of 546 tablet-based digital activities developed ad hoc for the program to reinforce multiple cognitive domains), motor activities (both adapted and light aerobic exercises) and behavioral suggestions (regarding sleeping times, daily naps, etc.), in addition to the monitoring of specific vital parameters already integrated in the TLM module.

This way, the Ability continuum-of-care platform works with a twofold scenario of use.

On the one hand, through the physician's portal, healthcare professionals are able to define the IRP according to individual clinical conditions of People With Dementia (PWD). They can set up the type and dose of motor and cognitive rehabilitation activities (e.g., establishing the sequential framing of cognitive activities reinforcing multiple domains of cognitive function, or defining the alternation between activity periods and pause periods), and the frequency of measurement of vital parameters. Moreover, they can support the rehabilitation process remotely, monitoring the progresses and, if needed, adapting the IRP to provide a day-by-day tailored intervention. They can also check the compliance with the at-home rehabilitation plan, contacting PWD and caregivers when appropriate, in order to adjust the intervention: for example, to improve motivation and to foster engagement in the care process.

On the other hand, through the user's portal, PWD and caregivers can access the IRP at home through a tablet application. On each day of intervention, after opening the user-friendly dashboard, PWD can see the cognitive and motor rehabilitation activities planned by the clinician for that day. A message on the dashboard appears more than once a week to recall them to measure the vital parameters, according to physician's recommendations. In the case of the Ability program, no tablet-based recalls were included regarding the Fitbit tracker, since participants were required to wear it continuously (24 h) throughout the intervention, except for very short interruptions to recharge it.

This way, PWD can take an active role in following the IRP at home with the prescribed sequence and timing of activities. At the same time, caregivers can monitor PWD's progresses, with the opportunity to be empowered with their autonomy in supporting the care process.

Based on the Ability platform and the scenario of use just outlined, it is herein described a use case that highlights how Carla, a person with cognitive disorders, succeeded in accomplishing the rehabilitation activities devised for his condition through the Ability continuum-of-care home program.

2.1 Heading the Target at the Right Pace: A Use Case of the Ability Continuum-of-Care Home Program

Carla is a 70-year-old scholar in Russian history still occasionally writing short papers and essays. In the last few years, she realized she had difficulties with her memory: she often forgot where she had left her home keys, or, if asked what she had eaten at lunch, she could no longer recollect it, even just few hours later. While she still was independent and autonomous in carrying out activities of daily living, with only minor difficulties in cooking a meal or arranging her outfit accurately, sleep disorders started to become more frequent. And writing her essays, especially in the morning as she was used to, turned out to be more demanding. Her husband was first puzzled, then worried, and, as these difficulties showed more and more often, he felt stressed for being unable to cope with them. After undergoing an extensive neuropsychological assessment and a clinical neurological evaluation, together with laboratory and imaging examinations, Carla was framed in the Mild Cognitive Impairment condition, a preclinical condition representing a risk factor for the development of AD. In view of this, clinicians also told Carla that several protective factors had been identified that may delay the onset of clinical AD. The multifactorial nature of AD indeed suggests that multicomponent interventions pointing at several risk factors simultaneously can generate optimal preventive effects. Concerning lifestyle-related risks, Carla was recommended to keep targeting a lifetime cognitive activity, combined with physical exercise, social stimulation, and appropriate nutritional guidance. She was therefore advised to accomplish several tasks according to the usual care protocol devised for outpatients of the Memory Clinic in the same preclinical condition. Regarding cognitive functioning, she received a workbook comprising paper and pencil cognitive activities to be performed at home for five days a week. She was also recommended to carry out a light aerobic motor activity every day (e.g., walking outdoor for about half an hour), to monitor blood pressure at least twice a week, and to keep her nutritional habits under control, shifting them towards Mediterranean diet options. She was then given a follow-up appointment after six months with the several professionals involved (physician, therapist, neuropsychologist). While being compliant with the program's task and recommendations in the first weeks, in the long run Carla started to feel less motivated in carrying them out. One day the weather was miserable and lying on the sofa reading with her cats was far more attracting to her than walking outdoors. Moreover, she felt that the progression of difficulty of cognitive activities (set independently of her cognitive resources) was often not in line with what she could (or could not) do. So, when activities were too easy for her, she sometimes performed also those prescribed for several days to come, while, if she perceived them too difficult, she simply gave them up. She also often forgot to monitor blood pressure. Timing and pacing of the several activities, and especially of physical exercises, were totally disrupted and, by the end of the second month, she felt disappointed and frustrated with the program, which she perceived as an objective she was virtually unable to pursue. At the six-month follow up, after clinical re-evaluation and neuropsychological assessments, a progression of impairment was detected, although she was still autonomous in her functional daily activities. In the meantime, among other front-edge neurorehabilitation research activities, the Memory Clinic was involved in a research project – the Ability project - envisioning a technology-enhanced concept of care for PWD, enabling smart continuity-of-care trajectories based on telemonitoring and telerehabilitation. About six months later, Carla was then invited at the Memory Clinic to join the Ability program for six consecutive weeks. At the beginning she was a bit nervous: she was not confident at all with tablets, and the kind of watch (the Fitbit tracker) she was asked to wear 24H seemed a bit too innovative and juvenile, compared to her feminine and traditional one. Anyway, together with her husband, she participated in the learning-by-doing training session of the telemonitoring devices and of the tablet activities, during which they became familiar with the dashboard that every day would deliver the cognitive, motor and monitoring activities that clinicians had set for her Individual Rehabilitation Plan. They went home with the Ability kit, that included: (a) the tablet for the delivery of the IRP, the memos for the monitoring of vital parameters and nutritional suggestions; (b) the Fitbit® Charge, to track motor and sleep activity; (c) a sphygmomanometer for the detection of blood pressure; (d) a pulse oximeter for the measurement of oxygen blood level and heart rate; (e) a scale for the detection of body weight; (f) the Telbios Station to send data collected from all the technological devices to the Ability platform.

During the six-week Ability program, Carla felt supported in her everyday rehabilitation tasks: the dashboard recalled her when to monitor vital parameters, while progression rules for increasing difficulty in cognitive activities fitted her resources in a way she perceived as well balanced. Watching the videos of exercises of adapted motor activity and doing them with her husband became a way to share their engagement in the process of care. Furthermore, turning on the tablet together every morning, checking activities, wearing a watch that tracked steps and sleep, and becoming progressively more confident in the interaction with the touch technology enhanced Carla's self-esteem, made her more active in conversations, and fostered her social interconnectedness through domains other than his "memory" difficulties.

From the clinician's perspective, setting Carla's Individual Rehabilitation Plan through the Ability physician's portal and meeting her and her husband for the training session required some extra effort, though still easily manageable, in the organization of the other clinical activities. The opportunity to monitor her vital motor activities from remote, how and when she slept, and how she coped with the dose and type of rehabilitation activities gave the physician a unique opportunity to elaborate on how the rehabilitation program impacted Carla's condition on a week-by-week basis. During the intervention, the clinician could modify the pacing of activities shifting the pause period in different days of the week, and, after noticing that a specific activity was often not accomplished, he could reset the progression rule for increasing difficulty, while asking her husband to support her in not giving up. Moreover, at the end of the program, he could combine the heterogeneous data (performance in cognitive and motor activities, sleep quality, and vital parameters metrics) collected by the Ability platform over the six weeks to give Carla an extensive and articulated feedback about "How it went". This way he could provide a robust basis to consolidate and/or to fix subsequent rehabilitation activities and to foster their therapeutic alliance in the continuum-of-care process.

Target, advantages/disadvantages with respect to current treatment options, technologies needed and main market indicators of the Ability program are briefly shown in Table 1.

Table 1. Target, key features with respect to current treatment options and main market indicators of the Ability program.

Primary users	People with MCI/PWD and formal (neurologist, therapist, neuropsychologist) and informal (e.g. spouse) caregivers
Secondary users	Service center
Target group size	Small
Market size	47.5 million people with dementia in 2015, 76 million estimated 2030
Current treatment/options	Paper and pencil cognitive activities or CD/DVD activities
Cost of current treatment/options	Quite low, considering the cost of consumables to deliver them
Advantages/disadvantages of current treatment/options	They cannot be personalized, they are not adaptable to user's cognitive resources, with risks of loss of motivation, they cannot be monitored remotely and modified until the next specialist visit
Who pays?	The user (in some cases the hospital)
Expected advantages/disadvantages compared to current treatment/options	It is possible to personalize the treatment, monitor it remotely, detect incompliance early, identify the motivation(s) and intervene timely to solve any issue. This will ensure PWD's and caregivers' active participation to the program's activities
From a user perspective, what needs to be resolved before applying the presented solution?	Proof of efficacy
Ethical issues	Privacy issues (data protection, exchange, etc.)

(*continued*)

Table 1. (*continued*)

Technologies needed	Telemonitoring platform and telemonitoring kit (set of devices and gateway)
Fields with shared benefits (synergies)	Serious gaming, wearable technologies, face-to-face multi-component rehabilitation
What is required to make this solution commercially viable?	Regulatory framework and reimbursement model
Incentive for industry, why would industry be interested?	The market is growing rapidly, as dementia is one of the main threats for people's health in the next years. So far there are few/no competitors on the market
Time to market	Short term (less than 3 years)

3 Concluding Remarks

Telerehabilitation has currently gained increasing attention as a rehabilitation strategy for PWD and people in the MCI condition, with evidence of positive effects for cognitive telerehabilitation comparable with face-to-face interventions [14]. At the same time, there are accumulating findings that multicomponent physical-cognitive interventions can improve cognitive status and indicators of brain health in MCI subjects [15, 16].

Based on the Ability platform, the Ability program was therefore designed and developed as an enhancement of usual care programs for people with MCI and PWD through technology. Its main innovation feature is that it promotes a comprehensive home-based continuity-of-care by the combination of: (a) a multicomponent (cognitive and motor activities) telerehabilitation intervention with (b) additional relevant care options like scheduled delivery of the IRP, telemonitoring of vital parameters, and tracking of physical activity. We devised to test its efficacy through a randomized two-treatment arms (Ability Program vs. Treatment As Usual) controlled clinical trial (ClinicalTrials.gov ID: NCT02746484NO; see [17] for full study protocol details), in line with the need to document the efficacy of technology-based interventions through high quality studies. Our expectation is that it will not only serve to mitigate AD progression, but will also benefit the subjective and psychological well-being of MCI subjects and people in early AD conditions, also through the design of the enabling role of technologies in line with the Positive Technology (PT) framework [18]. Such a framework views technologies as interfaces for personal experience, rather than as mere "devices", as in lay perspectives. This way, we envisage to empower social engagement within the care community of PWD and MCI subjects not just as a requirement for compliance with the scheduled activities, but also, being humans an ultrasocial and hyper-cooperative species [19], as the condition enabling the inter-subjective sharing of meaning among all the actors involved in the continuity-of-care process [20].

References

1. Byass, P.: A transition towards a healthier global population? Lancet **386**(10009), 2121–2122 (2015). https://doi.org/10.1016/S0140-6736(15)61476-3
2. Murray, C.J., et al.: Global, regional, and national disability-adjusted life years (DALYs) for 306 diseases and injuries and healthy life expectancy (HALE) for 188 countries, 1990–2013: quantifying the epidemiological transition. Lancet **386**(10009), 2145–2191 (2015). https://doi.org/10.1016/S0140-6736(15)61340-X
3. Winblad, B., et al.: Defeating Alzheimer's disease and other dementias: a priority for European science and society. Lancet Neurol. **15**, 455–532 (2015). https://doi.org/10.1016/S1474-4422(16)00062-4
4. Dubois, B., et al.: Preclinical Alzheimer's disease: definition, natural history, and diagnostic criteria. Alzheimers Dement **12**, 292–323 (2016). https://doi.org/10.1016/j.jalz.2016.02.002
5. Woods, B., Aguirre, E., Spector, A.E., Orrell, M.: Cognitive stimulation to improve cognitive functioning in people with dementia. Cochrane Database Syst. Rev. (2), CD005562 (2012). https://doi.org/10.1002/14651858.CD005562.pub2
6. Jean, L., Bergeron, M.È., Thivierge, S., Simard, M.: Cognitive intervention programs for individuals with mild cognitive impairment: systematic review of the literature. Am. J. Geriatr. Psychiat **18**, 281–296 (2010). https://doi.org/10.1097/JGP.0b013e3181c37ce9
7. García-Casal, J.A., Loizeau, A., Csipke, E., Franco-Martín, M., Perea-Bartolomé, M.V., Orrell, M.: Computer-based cognitive interventions for people living with dementia: a systematic literature review and meta-analysis. Aging Mental Health **21**, 454–467 (2016). https://doi.org/10.1080/13607863.2015.1132677
8. Theodoros, D., Russell, T., Latifi, R.: Telerehabilitation: current perspectives. Stud. Health Technol. Inform. **131**, 191–210 (2008)
9. Kairy, D., Lehoux, P., Vincent, C., Visintin, M.: A systematic review of clinical outcomes, clinical process, healthcare utilization and costs associated with telerehabilitation. Disabil. Rehabil. **31**, 427–447 (2009). https://doi.org/10.1080/09638280802062553
10. Dinesen, B., et al.: Personalized telehealth in the future: a global research agenda. J. Med. Internet Res. **18**, e53 (2016). https://doi.org/10.2196/jmir.5257
11. Martin, M., Clare, L., Altgassen, M., Cameron, H., Zehnder, F.: Cognition-based interventions for healthy older people and people with mild cognitive impairment. Cochrane Database Syst. Rev. (1) (2011). https://doi.org/10.1002/14651858.CD006220.pub2
12. Bahar-Fuchs, A., Clare, L., Woods, B.: Cognitive training and cognitive rehabilitation for mild to moderate Alzheimer's disease and vascular dementia. Cochrane Database Syst. Rev. (6) (2013). https://doi.org/10.1002/14651858.CD003260.pub2
13. Zygouris, S., Tsolaki, M.: Computerized cognitive testing for older adults: a review. Am. J. Alzheimers Dis. Other Demen. **30**, 13–28 (2015). https://doi.org/10.1177/1533317514522852
14. Cotelli, M., et al.: Cognitive telerehabilitation in mild cognitive impairment, Alzheimer's disease and frontotemporal dementia: a systematic review. J. Telemed. Telecare (2017). https://doi.org/10.1177/1357633X17740390
15. Baglio, F., et al.: Multistimulation group therapy in Alzheimer's disease promotes changes in brain functioning. Neurorehabilitation Neural Repair **29**, 13–24 (2015). https://doi.org/10.1177/1545968314532833
16. Maffei, L., et al.: Randomized trial on the effects of a combined physical/cognitive training in aged MCI subjects: the train the brain study. Sci. Rep. **7** (2017). https://doi.org/10.1038/srep39471

17. Realdon, O., et al.: Technology-enhanced multi-domain at home continuum of care program with respect to usual care for people with cognitive impairment: the Ability-TelerehABILITation study protocol for a randomized controlled trial. BMC Psychiatry **16**, 425 (2016). https://doi.org/10.1186/s12888-016-1132-y
18. Riva, G., Banos, R.M., Botella, C., Wiederhold, B.K., Gaggioli, A.: Positive technology: using interactive technologies to promote positive functioning. Cyberpsychol Behav. Soc. Netw. **15**, 69–77 (2012). https://doi.org/10.1089/cyber.2011.0139
19. Tomasello, M.: The Cultural Origins of Human Cognition. Harvard University Press, Cambridge (2009)
20. Wald, C.: Better together. Nature **531**, S14–S15 (2016). https://doi.org/10.1038/531S14a

The Use of 3D Body Scanner in Medicine and Psychology: A Narrative Review

Elisa Pedroli[1(✉)], Rossella Digilio[1], Cosimo Tuena[1],
Juan V. Durá-Gil[2], Franco Cernigliaro[3], Giuseppe Riva[1,4],
and Pietro Cipresso[1,4]

[1] Applied Technology for Neuro-Psychology Lab,
IRCCS Istituto Auxologico Italiano, Via L. Ariosto 13, 20145 Milan, MI, Italy
{e.pedroli, p.cipresso}@auxologico.it
digilio.rossella@gmail.com, cosimotuena@gmail.com
[2] Instituto de Biomecánica de Valencia, Universitat Politècnica de València,
46022 Valencia, Spain
juan.dura@ibv.upv.es
[3] U.O. Radiologia Ospedale San Luca IRCCS Istituto Auxologico Italiano,
Via L. Ariosto 13, 20145 Milan, MI, Italy
f.cernigliaro@auxologico.it
[4] Department of Psychology, Catholic University,
Largo Gemelli 1, 20100 Milan, MI, Italy
{giuseppe.riva, pietro.cipresso}@unicatt.it

Abstract. In this narrative review several articles that explain the application of 3D Body Scanner were analyzed. Among all published articles in the last 10 years only 14 met the inclusion criteria. There are several fields of application of this technology: Body shape and posture analysis, pediatrics, metrical analysis, and forensic medicine. The results indicate that 3D Body Scanner is a promising technology that could help clinicians and researchers to improve their work both in term of quality and time saving.

Keywords: 3D Body Scanner · Medicine · Psychology · Review

1 Introduction

Body scanning technology has been increasingly used in health research in the past years, extending its use from clothing industry. This technology allows researchers and clinicians to evaluate and obtain body shapes, sizes and great amount of data that can also be visualized thanks to an avatar. Traditionally, doctors have measured body parts by hand and use a sophisticated technology to produce 3D internal images of a patient's body. 3D body scanner can fill the gap and would enable clinicians to acquire complete 3D information of both inside and outside of patients. Three-dimensional body scanners used to capture anthropometric measurements are now becoming a common research tool because it is simultaneously efficient, cheap and provides virtually infinite number of measurements of every angle of the human body [1, 2].

© ICST Institute for Computer Sciences, Social Informatics and Telecommunications Engineering 2018
P. Cipresso et al. (Eds.): MindCare 2018, LNICST 253, pp. 74–83, 2018.
https://doi.org/10.1007/978-3-030-01093-5_10

Technically, 3D body scanner is a device that generates a 3-D "point cloud" from the subject's body a constellation of 100 000–200 000 points produced by the body's surface. These data are saved into a simple digital format and can easily be converted to the most common computer-aided design formats [3]. There are different kinds of body scanner techniques, such as laser scanning and white or structured light scanning. Besides, there are diverse type of scanners, including Human Solutions, Cyberware, Wicks and Wilson, Telmat or [TC]2 Body Measurement System [4]. Laser scanners sees light and couple charged device to detect light changes on surface, whereas white/structured light scanning requires projectors as a source of light and is faster than laser-based systems. This method uses stripes of white light on the subject and cameras to capture body shapes changes. Scanners adopt different techniques to extract data. For instance, Human Solutions scanner (e.g., Vitus Smart LC3) implements a system of laser triangulation, whilst Cyberware (e.g., Model WBX) using a patented Cyberware technology provides data thanks to four scanners. Wicks and Wilson (e.g., TriFormTM/TriBody) scanners use white light and eight cameras views to extract the shape. Telmat and its turbo flash 3D system SYMCAD (System for Measuring and Creating Anthropometric Database) utilizes structured light projected on the body and cameras.

Finally, [TC]2 Body Measurement System, based on white light system, provides a digital copy due to optical lenses. According to products reviewed on www.aniwaa.com the SYMCAD III (TELEMAT Industrie) utilizes near-IR structured light and takes only 1.5 s to scan the body, whereas the aforementioned scanners require 8–15 s. The Twinstant Mobile scanner allows to scan one to five bodies simultaneously as a result of the structured light and photogrammetry technologies. The cost varies on an average range of 10.000$–30.000$, as reported by www.aniwaa.com on the top 3D full body scanners chart. Despite differences in the way data are extracted, these scanners enable to create anthropometric models. Finally, avatar can be experienced by means of immersive technologies, such as motion capture and head mounted displays, allowing the user to have an illusion of embodiment in the avatar and the feeling of presence in the virtual environment [5].

2 Methods

2.1 Search Strategy

In 2007 two reviews about the clinical use of 3D body scanner were published [3, 6]. In one these articles authors described the Healthcare Applications of 3D Body Scanner in several field: epidemiology, diagnosis, treatment, and monitoring [6]. The other one is a literature survey of research work on HBS data segmentation and modeling [3]. That is the reason why the current article starts analyzing published article since then on.

To pursue this goal, a computer-based search in two databases was performed to retrieve relevant publications. Databases used for the search were: PubMed and Google Scholar. The search string was: "3D Body Scanner" AND ["Clinical" OR "Clinical Application"]. The articles were individually scanned to elaborate whether they fulfill the following inclusion criteria: (a) research article; (b) in the field of clinical application; and (c) published in English.

3 Results

In the current review, we aim to provide an initial review of the state-of-the-art studies from 2007 to 2017 focused on the use of 3D Body Scanner in medical and clinical application. In total, 14 studies met the inclusion criteria, which were critically reviewed, and are summarized in Table 1. In the following paragraphs, we reviewed the selected studies by dividing them according to the field of application of the technology: (1) body shape and posture analysis; (2) pediatric use; (3) metrical analysis; and (4) other applications.

Table 1. Characteristics of included studies

References	Scope	3D scanner type	Outcomes
Wells et al. [7]	Investigate the relation of shape and BMI and to examine associations between age, sex, and shape	3D whole body scanner, TC2 model	Relations between BMI and shape differed significantly between the sexes, particularly with regard to age. The inverse association between height and waist in men suggests either a genetic contribution or a link between early growth pattern and predisposition to obesity
Ashdown and Na [10]	Quantify the differences in posture and the differences in the amount of bilateral variation between the older and younger woman	Human Solutions VITUS/smart 3D body scanner	Of the 36 body taken measurements, 21 were significantly different between the two groups. The changes in linear measurements and angle measurement between the younger and older women indicate that there are significant differences in posture and in the amount of bilateral variation between the two groups. These differences will affect the fit of clothing
Bretschneider et al. [15]	Determine the precision and reproducibility of the body scanner for further applications	VITUS XXL 3D body scanner	The precision of the measurements of the circumferences of a truncated cone and a column was within 1 mm of the actual values (0.29%). These results show that the body scanner can accurately, precisely and reproducibly measure the circumference of objects and human body parts
Schloesser et al. [12]	Determine the BSA in healthy term neonates by 3D scanning	Prototype scanner constructed by 3D-Shape	3D scanning is an accurate and practical method to estimate BSA in newborns. One mathematical formula (Du Bois and Du Bois) showed a distinct underestimation of BSA compared to 3D scanning, the others an overestimation
Choi and Ashdown [1]	Test the accuracy and reliability of 3D measurements when taken on active body postures and analyze the change	Human Solutions VITUS XXL 3D whole body scanner	Results of calculating the body surface change rates for the lower body showed significant changes among the active postures. The analysis of the scan measurements demonstrated that the change in sitting posture generated the largest differences. These

(continued)

Table 1. (*continued*)

References	Scope	3D scanner type	Outcomes
	in lower body surface measurements		findings show the active changes in body measurements that occur with different postures for young women with hip measurements between 95 and 105 cm
Tomkinson and Shaw [16]	Used in the clinical setting as part of the examination process to assess musculoskeletal conditions	Vitus Smart 3D whole body scanner	Most standing postural measurements demonstrated good repeatability. However, head and neck postures demonstrated poor repeatability due to large random errors brought about by large postural errors. Overall, most of the error was due to postural error rather than technical error. The relatively small technical errors highlight that this 3D measurement process is generally repeatable, while the relatively large postural errors related to the head and neck suggest that these postures probably lack the precision to be clinically useful using this procedure
Daniell et al. [8]	Quantify shape differences associated with BMI	Vitus Smart 3D whole body scanner	There were nearly perfect correlations between WBV and BMI when analyzed by sex, with WBV increasing by about 3 l for every unit of BMI. While all segmental volumes increased significantly as BMI increased, the BMI-related patterns of increase varied among different body segments. Body shape changes due to variations in body volume could have important implications in a range of fields that currently use 1D anthropometric measurements that do not capture body shape differences in the same detail
Wells et al. [13]	Information on body size and shape used for interpretation of aspects of physiology in children, including nutritional status, cardio-metabolic risk and lung function	3D-PS	3D-PS is acceptable in children aged >5 years, though with current hardware/software, and body movement artefacts, approximately one third of scans may be unsuccessful. The technique had poorer technical success than manual measurements, and had poorer precision when the measurements were viable. Compared to manual measurements, 3D-PS showed modest average biases but acceptable limits of agreement for large surveys, and little evidence that bias varied substantially with size
Lee et al. [17]	Develop and validate a method for TBI treatment planning and compensator fabrication	Scan a RANDO™ phantom positioned in a TBI treatment	In vivo measurements for an end-to-end test showed that overall dose differences were within 5%. A technique for planning and fabricating a compensator for TBI treatment using a depth camera equipped tablet and a 3D printer was demonstrated to be sufficiently accurate to be considered for further investigation

(*continued*)

Table 1. (*continued*)

References	Scope	3D scanner type	Outcomes
Ng et al. [14]	Investigation for clinically relevant direct anthropometrics and body composition measurement	3D surface scan	Strong associations of waist and hip circumference to tape-measured values, body surface area to the Du Bois model and body volumes to DXA volume estimates. 3D surface scanners offer precise and stable automated measurements of body shape and composition. Software updates may be needed to resolve measurement biases resulting from landmark positioning discrepancies
Serino et al. [9]	Representation of the body, in terms of body size estimations, with VR (Virtual Reality) body swapping	Size Stream 3D body scanner	After participants embodied a virtual body with a skinny belly (independently of the type of visuo-tactile stimulation), there was an update of the stored representation of the body: participants reported a decrease in the ratio between estimated and actual body measures for most of the body parts considered. Scanner is used to collect measures
Liu et al. [2]	Develop estimation formulae for the total human body volume (BV) of adult males using anthropometric measurements based on a 3D scanning technique	Three-dimensional (3D) scanner	The linear model based on human weight was recommended as the most optimal due to its simplicity and high efficiency. The proposed estimation formulae are valuable for estimating total body volume in circumstances in which traditional underwater weighing or air displacement plethysmography is not applicable or accessible
Cornelissen et al. [11]	Body image distortion in Anorexia Nervosa	Size Stream 3D body scanner	Women who are in treatment for ANSD show an over-estimation of body size which rapidly increases as their own BMI does. By contrast, the women acting as healthy controls can accurately estimate their body size irrespective of their own BMI
Kottner et al. [18]	Forensic imaging investigations	VirtoScan: mobile, multi-camera rig based on close-range photogrammetry	A surface model comparison between the high-resolution output from our in-house standard and a high-resolution model from the multi-camera rig showed a mean surface deviation of 0.36 mm for the whole body scan and 0.13 mm for a second comparison of a detailed section of the scan. The use of the multi-camera rig reduces the acquisition time for whole-body surface documentations in medicolegal examinations and provides a low-cost 3D surface scanning alternative for forensic investigations

3.1 Body Shape and Posture Analysis

Four articles are categorized into this area. In particular, two of them connect the analysis of the body scan with the Body Mass Index (BMI) [7, 8]. This index is a common indicator in many medical fields. Developing a system to calculate precisely BMI could be an interesting research topic.

Wells and colleagues [7] investigated the relation of shape and BMI, examining associations between age, sex, and shape in a group of 9617 adults. They used a 3D Body Scanner TC2 model ([TC]2, Cary, NC) for the acquisitions of the shape, body girths and their ratios; authors also collect weight and height to obtain BMI. The results of this wide study are several and specific for age and sex. While in men BMI was associated with chest and waist girths; in women, the BMI is related to the measures of hips and bust. These associations are more valid in early adulthood and they tend to decrease with age. In women waist girths increase with age while thigh girths decreased; in men, all the measures remained stable. The authors also reported that after adjustment for other girths, particularly for men, waist was significantly and inversely associated with height [7].

The second article tried to quantify differences in body shape among people with different BMI [8]. With that aim, they used the Vitus Smart whole-body scanner (Human Solutions, Kaiserslautern, Germany) and the data analysis was made using ScanWorx Editor and translated into a readable format for use in the CySlice v.3.4 (Headus, Perth, Australia) measurement extraction software. The authors analyzed eight segmental volumes: Neck, Shoulder, Elbow, Thorax, Abdominal, Hip and Knee in 340 young adults. The authors showed that while both segmental volumes and BMI increased significantly, the BMI-related patterns of increase varied among the different body parts analyzed. Accordingly, authors who underline the importance of under-standing this relationship in order to develop a Body Volume Index or Surface Area Index may provide a tool that is more strongly associated with shape changes than BMI [8].

Another research group uses a 3D body scanner technology in order to obtain much precise measures, as well as to calculate BMI [9]. The authors aimed to investigate if an innovative virtual reality (VR) system for the body swapping illusion can be an effective for modifying the enduring memory of the body. Results showed that after the illusion there was an update of the stored representation of the body; participants reported a decrease in the ratio between estimated and actual body measures for most of the body parts considered. These findings provide first evidence that VR body swapping can induce a change in the memory of the body. The use of the Size Stream 3D Body Scanner allows the researcher to obtain a more precise measurement of the subjects' body to be compared with the other data [9].

Ashdown and colleague [10] use 3D body scanner to analyzed posture to assess the change over the age in a sample of women. These changes have been documented in many studies and in this study these results are validate. Using 3D measurements, the authors try to quantify the differences in posture and the differences in the amount of bilateral variation between the older and younger women. An important result emerged indicating an asymmetrical body configuration for the group of older women compared to the young one. The authors recorded 36 body measurements and find that 21 were significantly different between the two groups of women. These results are important both for the clothing industries and the health field [10].

In the last article of this section authors [11] used 3D Body Scanner to obtain an avatar of the patients. The authors modified the body shape of the avatars with the aim of quantifying over-estimation of the body in anorexic patients and healthy women. Before the implementation of 3D Body Scanner and CGI technology this process would not have been possible; the authors combine these two tools to create an innovative system. The results demonstrate the great utility of the system proposed to create personalized avatars of patients to assess their body image perception [11].

3.2 Pediatric Use

Two articles analyzed the possible use of the 3D Body Scanner with children in two different age sample.

In the first article authors [12] try to determinate the Body Surface Area (BSA) in healthy term and near-term neonates using the 3D body scanner technology. The authors developed and use a prototype constructed especially for the study by 3D-Shape, Erlangen, Germany because no commercial scanners are suitable to use with neonates. On 209 infants analyzed, only 53 acceptable images are collected. Despite this, the authors conclude that 3D scanning is an accurate and practical method to estimate BSA in neonates because allow to obtain individual day to day measures [12].

Wells and colleagues analyzed the Acceptability, Precision and Accuracy of 3D Photonic Scanning obtained with NX16 instrumentation ([TC]2, Cary, North Carolina) [13]. They collect measures manually and by 3D-PS in a multi-ethnic sample of 1484 child. Manual measurements were successful in all cases. Although successful scans were only obtained in 70.7%, mostly because of the movement of children. Compared to manual measurements, 3D body scanner measures had modest average biases but acceptable limits of agreement for large surveys, and little evidence that bias varied substantially with size.

3.3 Metrical Analysis

Measurement repeatability has important decision-making implications for clinicians and researchers when assessing individuals.

In their research Ng and colleagues [14] investigated if 3D body surface scanners can provide interested clinically direct anthropometrics and body composition estimates. They analyzed thirty-nine healthy adults with different age, sex and BMI with a Fit3D Proscanner (Fit3D Inc., Redwood City, CA, USA), dual energy X-ray absorptiometry (DXA), air displacement plethysmography (ADP), and tape measurements. The authors concluded that 3D surface scanners offer precise and stable automated measurements of body shape and composition. In particular, the use of 3D surface scanning is an accurate, precise and automated substitute to other methods such as measuring tape, ADP and DXA [14].

In the second paper analyzed by the authors [15], they try to establish how the measurements obtained with VITUS XXL 3D body scanner are precise and reproducible. Bretschneider and colleagues compared geometric shapes and human body parts using a measuring tape and the body scanner. Accordingly with the expectations, the results show that the measurements obtained with 3D body scanner are accurate, precise, and reproducible both for the circumference of objects and human body parts [15].

Choi and colleagues [1] used 3D scans to measure and analyze lower body measurement change for various active body positions. They compared the measurements from each posture to a standing posture and tested the reliability of the 3D measurements on active postures. Also, authors compare 3D scan measurements using virtual tools on the computer screen with traditional manual anthropometric measurements. The measurement obtained from 3D scans constitutes a reliable and appropriate method for comparative measurements between active body positions, contrary to standard anthropometric methods [1].

Four articles about the accuracy of the 3D body scanner measurement were published in 2013 by Tomkinson and Shaw [16]. The aims of the study were to quantify both the repeatability of direct measurements of standing posture as well as the characteristics of the postural and technical errors. During the process emerged that most of the error arose from postural error rather than technical ones. Accordingly, the authors concluded that 3D measurement process is repeatable, while the problem was related to the head and neck postures required during the process [16].

The last study of this section aimed to develop estimation formulae for the total human body volume (BV) of adult males [2]. To do that, the authors used measurements collected through a 3D body scanner technique. A regression analysis of BV based on four key measurements was conducted and eight total models of human BV show that the predicted results fitted by the regression models. So, the proposed estimation formulae are useful in estimating total body volume instead of classical measurement techniques [2].

3.4 Other Applications

Another interesting application of 3D body scanner technology is presented by Lee and colleagues [17]. They studied an innovative system to create a compensator in order to allow a better and uniform distribution throughout the body during a session of total body irradiation (TBI). Using depth-sensing cameras (Project Tango Developer Kit, Google, Inc., Mountain View, CA, USA) and 3D printing authors create a tablet to scan the body and elaborate and sending the data to the printing. The characteristics of the process and of the compensator allow to consider this prototype an interesting subject for future investigations [17].

3D body scanning techniques could be used profitably also in the forensic field. Kottner and colleagues [18] present an application of VirtoScan, a mobile, multi-camera rig based on close-range photogrammetry, for this kind of analysis. The aim is to add this measurements with other post-mortem investigations like post-mortem computed tomography (PMCT) and post-mortem magnetic resonance imaging (PMMR). The system presented allows to dramatically reduce the acquisition time for the whole-body surface during the medicolegal examinations providing a detailed low-cost 3D surface scanning for forensic investigations.

4 Discussion

Within the analyzed articles, it emerged that 3D body Scanner is a valid instrument that allows to research and clinicians to acquire easily a lot of information about their patients.

The fields of application in medicine for this technology are many and in each of these the implementation of the scanner can bring benefits.

The scanner was used to took measures in several research papers, most of the time to obtain precision and saving time, both for adults and children, even neonates. On the one hand, the possibility of obtaining several body indicators in a short amount of time encourage the researcher to use this toll. On the other hand, the cost of the technology and problem of space could not entice the clinicians to use the scanner.

Despite this, the use with children requires to overcome some problems, especially regarding the movement of the sample. Realistically, most of these limitations could be addressed through further technological development, turning this technology into a gold standard in the pediatric analysis.

The analysis performed to control the stability and the accuracy of the 3D body scanner technology reported very interesting and positive results. All the articles report that this tool is much more precise, fast and accurate than classical measurement systems.

Finally, the advantages of the use of the 3D body scanner overcome the problems and limitations identified in the analysis. Thus, this technology constitutes a useful tool for several applications in medicine and the clinical field.

Acknowledgments. The present work was supported by the European funded project "Body-Pass" – API-ecosystem for cross-sectorial exchange of 3D personal data (H2020-779780).

References

1. Choi, S., Ashdown, S.P.: 3D body scan analysis of dimensional change in lower body measurements for active body positions. Text. Res. J. **81**(1), 81–93 (2011)
2. Liu, X., et al.: Estimation of human body volume (BV) from anthropometric measurements based on three-dimensional (3D) scan technique. Aesthet. Plastic Surg. **41**(4), 971–978 (2017)
3. Werghi, N.: Segmentation and modeling of full human body shape from 3-D scan data: a survey. IEEE Trans. Syst. Man Cybern. Part C (Appl. Rev.) **37**(6), 1122–1136 (2007)
4. Apeagyei, P.R.: Application of 3D body scanning technology to human measurement for clothing Fit. Change **4**(7), 58–68 (2010)
5. Kilteni, K., Groten, R., Slater, M.: The sense of embodiment in virtual reality. Presence: Teleoper. Virtual Env. **21**(4), 373–387 (2012)
6. Treleaven, P., Wells, J.: 3D body scanning and healthcare applications. Computer. **40**(7), 28–34 (2007)
7. Wells, J.C., Treleaven, P., Cole, T.J.: BMI compared with 3-dimensional body shape: the UK National Sizing Survey. Am. J. Clin. Nutrition **85**(2), 419–425 (2007)

8. Daniell, N., Olds, T., Tomkinson, G.: Volumetric differences in body shape among adults with differing body mass index values: an analysis using three-dimensional body scans. Am. J. Hum. Biol. **26**(2), 156–163 (2014)
9. Serino, S., et al.: Virtual reality body swapping: a tool for modifying the allocentric memory of the body. Cyberpsychol. Behav. Soc. Netw. **19**(2), 127–133 (2016)
10. Ashdown, S.P., Na, H.: Comparison of 3-D body scan data to quantify upper-body postural variation in older and younger women. Cloth. Tex. Res. J. **26**(4), 292–307 (2008)
11. Cornelissen, K.K., et al.: Body size estimation in women with anorexia nervosa and healthy controls using 3D avatars. Sci. Rep. **7**(1), 15773 (2017)
12. Schloesser, R., et al.: Three-dimensional body scanning: a new method to estimate body surface area in neonates. Neonatology **100**(3), 260–264 (2011)
13. Wells, J.C., et al.: Acceptability, precision and accuracy of 3D photonic scanning for measurement of body shape in a multi-ethnic sample of children aged 5-11 years: the SLIC study. PLoS ONE **10**(4), e0124193 (2015)
14. Ng, B., et al.: Clinical anthropometrics and body composition from 3D whole-body surface scans. Eur. J. Clin. Nutrition **70**, 1265 (2016)
15. Bretschneider, T., et al.: Validation of the body scanner as a measuring tool for a rapid quantification of body shape. Skin Res. Technol. **15**(3), 364–369 (2009)
16. Tomkinson, G.R., Shaw, L.G.: Quantification of the postural and technical errors in asymptomatic adults using direct 3D whole body scan measurements of standing posture. Gait Posture **37**(2), 172–177 (2013)
17. Lee, M.Y., et al.: A depth-sensing technique on 3D-printed compensator for total body irradiation patient measurement and treatment planning. Med. Phys. **43**(11), 6137–6144 (2016)
18. Kottner, S., et al.: VirtoScan - a mobile, low-cost photogrammetry setup for fast post-mortem 3D full-body documentations in x-ray computed tomography and autopsy suites. Forensic Sci. Med. Pathol. **13**(1), 34–43 (2017)

The Contribution of Allocentric Impairments to the Cognitive Decline in Alzheimer's Disease

Silvia Serino[1,2(✉)], Francesca Morganti[3], Desirèe Colombo[4],
and Giuseppe Riva[1,2]

[1] Applied Technology for Neuro-Psychology Lab,
IRCCS Istituto Auxologico Italiano, Via Magnasco, 2, 20149 Milan, Italy
s.serino@auxologico.it
[2] Department of Psychology, Università Cattolica del Sacro Cuore,
Largo Gemelli, 1, 20100 Milan, Italy
[3] Department of Human and Social Sciences, University of Bergamo,
Piazzale S. Agostino 2, 24129 Bergamo, BG, Italy
[4] Department of Basic Psychology, Clinic and Psychobiology,
Universitat Jaume I, Av. Sos Baynat, s/n, 12071 Castellón, Spain

Abstract. An early decline in navigation abilities is one of the first sign of Alzheimer's Disease (AD). More specifically, it has been suggested that allocentric impairments contribute significantly to this pathological decline. In this vein, the objective of the current work was to investigate the contribution of different spatial abilities involved in navigation (including allocentric ones) to the cognitive decline. Thirty elderly participated in the study, divided into two groups: Fifteen cognitively healthy aged individuals and fifteen individuals with AD. Our results showed that patients with AD performed significantly poorer in almost all tests evaluating spatial abilities in comparison to cognitively healthy aged individuals. Interestingly, we found that the allocentric abilities were the only significant predictor of the cognitive decline. Overall, these results suggested the primary role of allocentric impairments in contributing to the cognitive pathological decline.

Keywords: Allocentric abilities · Spatial navigation · Virtual Reality
Alzheimer's Disease

1 Introduction

Getting back home using a new route, visiting a museum in a new city, finding our car in a large parking lot: These are very common daily life situations in which spatial abilities play a key role. Spatial navigation, i.e. the ability of finding and tracking a path from one place to another [1, 2] is crucial ability needing the contribution of different cognitive abilities. Above all, it requires the ability to maintain an internal representation of the external environment, which includes the storage of spatial information in short and long-term memory collected from different sensory systems, and the manipulation of these representations for different navigational purposes [1]. A robust body of studies indicated that the cognitive profile of Alzheimer's Disease (AD) is

© ICST Institute for Computer Sciences, Social Informatics and Telecommunications Engineering 2018
P. Cipresso et al. (Eds.): MindCare 2018, LNICST 253, pp. 84–91, 2018.
https://doi.org/10.1007/978-3-030-01093-5_11

severely characterized by early spatial navigation impairments [3–8]. Moreover, spatial impairments contribute seriously to the initial pathological decline observed in individuals suffering from Mild Cognitive Impairment (MCI), i.e. a transitional state between the physiological and the pathological aging, marked by a slight deterioration of cognitive abilities, especially involving memory [9]. Interestingly, AD and MCI patients show profound impairments involving both allocentric (i.e., a spatial reference frame based on object-to-object relations) and egocentric (i.e., a spatial reference frame based on self-to-object relations), with a major degeneration in using allocentric strategies [6]. Recently, Laczó and co-workers [10] found in a sample of 108 older adults (53 cognitively normal individuals and 55 individuals with amnestic MCI) that spatial navigation deficits may be distinguished from deficits occurring in other cognitive domains, thus suggesting the importance of a prompt testing of this cognitive ability to early detect suspicious cases of cognitive decline. Allocentric impairments are the core spatial difficulties in individuals suffering from AD and MCI [4, 6], since neurodegenerative processes primarily involve the medial temporal lobes and related areas [11–15]. Indeed, allocentric deficits could lead to great navigational impairments, preventing the patient from maintaining a coherent "cognitive map" of the external environment [16, 17]. A decline in spatial abilities characterizes also normal aging, with an impact in the ability to retain information [18–20] and use them for navigating in surrounding environment [4, 21]. In particular, this decline in spatial abilities concerns the ability to store allocentric representations, and a growing body of studies indicated that it starts around the 60 years of age, when there is a concurrent deterioration of medial temporal lobes [22–25]. For instance, Gazova and co-workers [22] used a human adapted version of the Morris Water Maze Test to investigate differences in allocentric, egocentric and learning abilities between younger and older participants. Findings pointed out a specific deficit in allocentric retrieval in older individuals, but no impairments in the other spatial abilities investigated. Starting from these premises, the aim of the current study was to conduct a systematic investigation of spatial abilities in a sample of patients suffering from AD and in a matched control group of cognitively healthy elderly individuals, focusing on the relation between spatial abilities involved in navigation (including the allocentric ones) and the general cognitive functioning.

2 Methods

2.1 Participants

Thirty elderly subjects participated in the study, divided into two groups: 15 elderly suffering from probable AD ("AD group") and 15 cognitively healthy elderly individuals (CG, control group). AD patients were recruited from a social senior centre located in Lombardy (Italy) from those referred as meeting the NINCDS-ARDRA criteria for probable AD [26]. These patients were further evaluated with the Milan Overall Dementia Scale [27] and only those having a score under 85.5 were included in the study. AD group had a mean score at the Mini-Mental State Examination - MMSE [28] of 22.11 (SD = 2.12). The cognitively healthy elderly individuals, who were recruited from a panel of volunteers without neurological or psychiatric disorders (evaluated with a brief interview), had a mean score of MMSE [28] of 28.79 (SD = 1.84). The AD group was composed of 11 women and 4 men, while the CG included 12 women and 3 men [(χ^2 = 0.186(1); p = 0.666)]. The mean age for the AD group was 86.73 (3.97), with a mean years of education of 7.33 (SD = 1.91), while the mean age for the CG was 83.53 (5.62), with a mean years of education of 5.87 (SD = 2.92). There were no significant differences between the two groups concerning neither age [t(28) = 1.801; p = 0.082)] or education [t(28) = −1.625; p = 0.115)].

2.2 Spatial Assessment

In order to examine the various aspects of spatial navigation, we carried out a comprehensive assessment of spatial abilities in terms of short and long-term spatial memory [the Corsi Block Test [29, 30] in both its version Corsi Span and Corsi Supraspan], visuo-spatial abilities [Judgment of Line Orientation - JLO [31], navigation abilities [Money's Standardized Road Map Test [32], and egocentric mental rotation abilities [the Manikin Test [33]. As concerns the assessment of allocentric abilities, a Virtual Reality (VR)-based procedure was employed (for a detailed description, please see [34, 35]) After an initial training in the use of VR technology, elderly individuals were invited to enter in a virtual room which included only two objects (i.e., a plant and a stone) and an arrow drawn on the floor, which pointed to the North (i.e., *encoding phase*). Elderly were asked to memorize the position of the plant, which was positioned at different points in the virtual environment. The entire procedure was repeated across four randomized trials. In the first trial, the stone was located on the north and the plant on the east side of the environment, while in the second one the stone was still located on the north, but the plant was on the west. In the third and in the fourth trial, instead, the stone was on the south, whereas the plant was posited on the east side for the third trial and on the west side during the fourth one. Successively, participants were asked to retrieve the position of the object they had previously memorized on a map – a full aerial view of the virtual room (i.e., *retrieval phase*). This task was used as a measure of the ability to retrieve a stored allocentric representation. The accuracy of spatial location was the dependent variable: 0 = no answer or poor answer (for example, choosing the same side of the retrieval point (i.e. the North); 1 = correct answer. To obtain a composite score, we also added up the scores obtained from each trial (namely, we obtained an index measuring the allocentric abilities, "Allocentric Abilities"). This VR-based procedure was developed using the software NeuroVirtual 3D [36].

2.3 Procedure

After administering the Mini-Mental State Examination to obtain a picture of the general cognitive functioning, the comprehensive assessment of different spatial abilities involved in navigation was delivered (i.e., Money's Standardized Road Map Test, Manikin Test, Corsi, Judgment of Line Orientation) by an expert neuropsychologist. As regards the VR-based task for measuring the allocentric abilities, participants were invited to sit comfortably in front of a portable computer (ACER ASPIRE with CPU Intel® Core™i5 and graphic processor Nvidia GeForce GT 540 M, 1024 × 768 resolution). A gamepad was used to explore and interact with the virtual room (Logitech

Rumble F510). The training phase was delivered to allow participants interacting autonomously with VR (approximately two-five minutes). Then, the VR-based task started.

3   Results

AD patients, relative to CG, displayed significantly poorer long-term, visuo-spatial and egocentric mental rotation skills, with greater deficiencies also in the "allocentric retrieval" (Table 1). In other words, AD patients performed significantly poorer in respect to cognitively healthy elderly controls in most of the spatial abilities investigated.

Table 1. Performance of participants suffering from Alzheimer's Disease (AD group) and of cognitively healthy elderly controls on spatial abilities. Values are shown as mean (SD)

	AD group	CG	t	df	p^1	d^2
Corsi Block Test-Span	4.217 (0.706)	4.617 (0.674)	−1.587	28	0.124	0.57
Corsi Block Test-Supraspan	5.001 (2.959)	9.904 (7.124)	−2.052	18.69	0.024	0.89
Manikin Test	20.60 (4.421)	25.53 (4.912)	−2.891	28	0.007	1.05
Judgment of Line Orientation	9.27 (5.946)	17.227 (6.273)	−3.585	28	0.001	1.30
Money Road Map	18.23 (4.809)	21.40 (4.748)	−1.872	28	0.072	0.66
Allocentric Abilities	1.933 (0.799)	2.733 (0.799)	−2.743	28	0.011	1.00

[1] p-value; [2] effect size (d > 0.80 can be considered as a high effect size).

A linear regression analysis was carried out to investigate the extent to which scores on the spatial assessment might contribute to the cognitive decline, using scores of MMSE (as a measure of cognitive functioning) as dependent measure. All independent variables were entered singularly into the model using the 'enter' method. Findings showed that spatial assessment was able to predict the pathological decline [$R^2 = 0.546$; $F_{(6; 23)} = 4.61823$; $p = 0.003$). However, results showed that the allocentric abilities were the only significant predictor of cognitive functioning (see Table 2).

Table 2. Summary table of the regression analysis with spatial abilities as predictors and MMSE as dependent variable. Beta unstandardized coefficient are reported.

	B	SE	t	p
Corsi Block Test-Span	0.649	0.827	0.784	0.441
Corsi Block Test-Supraspan	0.223	0.119	1.879	0.073
Manikin Test	0.103	0.162	0.638	0.530
Judgment of Line Orientation	0.074	0.099	0.747	0.462
Money Road Map	−0.101	0.145	−0.696	0.494
Allocentric Abilities	1.983	0.698	2.840	0.009

4 Discussion

An abundant body of studies indicated that spatial abilities impairments are present in the cognitive profile of both normal and pathological aging. This means that a premature deterioration of navigational abilities, and in particular a deficit in the ability to encode and store allocentric information for navigating in the surrounding environment, represents one of the first hallmarks of Alzheimer's Disease (AD). However, as previously discussed, allocentric difficulties characterize the cognitive status of cognitively healthy aged people (for a review, see [37]). In this view, the current study was aimed to investigate the contribution of allocentric impairments to general cognitive decline, measured with the Mini-Mental State Examination (MMSE).

Our results showed that patients with AD performed significantly poorer in almost all tests evaluating spatial abilities in comparison to the cognitively healthy aged individuals, including the ability to retrieve allocentric representations (measured with the VR-based task [34, 35]). Moreover, we found that the allocentric abilities were the only significant predictors of cognitive functioning (as measured with the MMSE), thus suggesting its primary role in predicting the cognitive decline.

First of all, these results are in line with literature about spatial navigational deficits early manifested in AD [3–7]. Interestingly, our results did not suggest the presence of a significant difference between the two groups in the short-term spatial memory and general navigation abilities, but in other more specific spatial abilities that are essential for a successful navigation, such us the visuo-spatial and the egocentric mental rotation skills. Our findings are also in line with recent studies suggesting early impairments in crucial spatial abilities in AD, such as the perspective taking abilities [38–40]. Perspective taking (i.e., the ability to take different viewpoints in space) requires a manipulation centred on one's own body and it is traditionally distinguished from the object-based manipulation [41], where the observer remains mentally fixed and is asked to mentally rotate the object. Moreover, from our results emerged a central role of allocentric impairments among other spatial abilities in predicting the general cognitive functioning of participants and, therefore, the pathological cognitive decline of AD patients. Beyond the hippocampal decline observed in both normal aging and AD, allocentric and egocentric frames show different underlying cognitive mechanisms. Consistently with literature [8, 42–46], our results supported the idea that the allocentric decline may be a disease-specific marker of pathological degeneration. More interestingly, it is possible that this deficit in egocentric frame may be linked to another spatial ability involved in navigation, namely the capacity in the allocentric-to-egocentric switching or synchronization [35, 40, 47]. Indeed, it is suggested that egocentric short-term representations are transformed in long-term allocentric ones for storage; then, when there is retrieval cue, allocentric representations are transformed again in an egocentric format, which is more useful for navigation [48, 49]. In this perspective, the cognitive profile of AD may be marked by a very early deficit in the storage of an allocentric representation, combined with another early impairment in the ability to retrieve this representation and transform it an egocentric format with a synchronized egocentric direction useful for an effective orientation in the environment [16, 17, 47].

These results surely open future possibilities for new research studies; however it is crucial to acknowledge some limitations. First of all, the two samples recruited for this study are rather small, although they were well-matched for the main sociodemographic characteristics. However, although the between-group difference is not statistically significant, it is noteworthy to note that the healthy sample had mean years of education of 5.87, much lower than AD patients. Moreover, we could not deeply investigate the cognitive mechanisms involved in allocentric elaborations, as we did not assess participants for executive functions or attentional abilities. Although these findings are promising and may stimulate further research in this field, future studies should investigate the potential value of different spatial abilities as cognitive diagnostic markers in AD.

Acknowledgement. This work was partially supported by the Italian funded project "High-end and Low-End Virtual Reality Systems for the Rehabilitation of Frailty in the Elderly" (PE-2013-02355948), by the research project Tecnologia Positiva e Healthy Aging (Positive Technology and Healthy Aging) (Grant D.3.2., 2014) and by the research project "Ageing and Healthy Living: A Human Centered Approach in Research and innovation as Source of Quality Life", funded by Fondazione Cariplo within the 2014.

References

1. Wolbers, T., Hegarty, M.: What determines our navigational abilities? Trends Cogn. Sci. **14** (3), 138–146 (2010)
2. Gallistel, C.R.: The Organization of Learning. MIT Press, Cambridge (1990)
3. Allison, S.L., et al.: Spatial navigation in preclinical Alzheimer's disease. J. Alzheimer's DISEASE 1–14 (2016, preprint)
4. Lithfous, S., Dufour, A., Després, O.: Spatial navigation in normal aging and the prodromal stage of Alzheimer's disease: insights from imaging and behavioral studies. Ageing Res. Rev. **12**(1), 201–213 (2013)
5. Gazova, I., et al.: Spatial navigation—a unique window into physiological and pathological aging. Front. Aging Neurosci. **4**, 16 (2012)
6. Serino, S., et al.: The role of egocentric and allocentric abilities in Alzheimer's disease: a systematic review. Ageing Res. Rev. **16**, 32–44 (2014)
7. Boccia, M., et al.: Neural underpinnings of the decline of topographical memory in mild cognitive impairment. Am. J. Alzheimer's Disease Other Dementias (2016). https://doi.org/10.1177/1533317516654757
8. Weniger, G., et al.: Egocentric and allocentric memory as assessed by virtual reality in individuals with amnestic mild cognitive impairment. Neuropsychologia **49**(3), 518–527 (2011)
9. Petersen, R.C.: Mild cognitive impairment as a diagnostic entity. J. Intern. Med. **256**(3), 183–194 (2004)
10. Laczó, J., et al.: Exploring the contribution of spatial navigation to cognitive functioning in older adults. Neurobiol. Aging **51**, 67–70 (2017)
11. Braak, H., Braak, E.: Neuropathological stageing of Alzheimer-related changes. Acta Neuropathol. **82**(4), 239–259 (1991)
12. Braak, H., Braak, E.: Evolution of the neuropathology of Alzheimer's disease. Acta Neurol. Scand. **94**(S165), 3–12 (1996)

13. Alafuzoff, I., et al.: Staging of neurofibrillary pathology in Alzheimer's disease: a study of the BrainNet Europe Consortium. Brain Pathol. **18**(4), 484–496 (2008)
14. Dickson, D.W.: The pathogenesis of senile plaques. J. Neuropathol. Exp. Neurol. **56**(4), 321–339 (1997)
15. Thal, D.R., et al.: Sequence of Aβ-protein deposition in the human medial temporal lobe. J. Neuropathol. Exp. Neurol. **59**(8), 733–748 (2000)
16. Serino, S., Riva, G.: Getting lost in Alzheimer's disease: a break in the mental frame syncing. Med. Hypotheses **80**(4), 416–421 (2013)
17. Serino, S., Riva, G.: What is the role of spatial processing in the decline of episodic memory in Alzheimer's disease? The "mental frame syncing" hypothesis. Front. Aging Neurosci. **6**, 33 (2014)
18. Wolbers, T., Dudchenko, P.A., Wood, E.R.: Spatial memory - a unique window into healthy and pathological aging. Front. Aging Neurosci. **6**, 35 (2014)
19. Iachini, I., et al.: Visuospatial memory in healthy elderly, AD and MCI: a review. Curr. Aging Sci. **2**(1), 43–59 (2009)
20. Nemmi, F., Boccia, M., Guariglia, C.: Does aging affect the formation of new topographical memories? Evidence from an extensive spatial training. Neuropsychol. Dev. Cogn. B Aging Neuropsychol. Cogn. **24**(1), 29–44 (2017)
21. Moffat, S.D.: Aging and spatial navigation: what do we know and where do we go? Neuropsychol. Rev. **19**(4), 478–489 (2009)
22. Gazova, I., et al.: Spatial navigation in young versus older adults. Front. Aging Neurosci. **5**, 94 (2013)
23. Ruggiero, G., D'Errico, O., Iachini, T.: Development of egocentric and allocentric spatial representations from childhood to elderly age. Psychol. Res. **80**(2), 259–272 (2016)
24. Montefinese, M., et al.: Age-related effects on spatial memory across viewpoint changes relative to different reference frames. Psychol. Res. **79**(4), 687–697 (2015)
25. Wiener, J.M., Kmecova, H., de Condappa, O.: Route repetition and route retracing: effects of cognitive aging. Spatial memory – a unique window into healthy and pathological ageing (2015)
26. McKhann, G., et al.: Clinical diagnosis of Alzheimer's disease report of the NINCDS-ADRDA Work Group* under the auspices of Department of Health and Human Services Task Force on Alzheimer's disease. Neurology **34**(7), 939 (1984)
27. Brazzelli, M., et al.: A neuropsychological instrument adding to the description of patients with suspected cortical dementia: the Milan overall dementia assessment. J. Neurol. Neurosurg. Psychiatr. **57**(12), 1510–1517 (1994)
28. Folstein, M.F., Robins, L.N., Helzer, J.E.: The mini-mental state examination. Arch. Gener. Psychiatr. **40**(7), 812 (1983)
29. Corsi, P.M.: Human memory and the medial temporal region of the brain. ProQuest Information & Learning (1973)
30. Spinnler, H., Tognoni, G.: Standardizzazione e taratura italiana di test neuropsicologici. Ital. J. Neurol. Sci. **6**(8), 1–119 (1987)
31. Benton, A.L., Varney, N.R., des Hamsher, K.: Visuospatial judgment: a clinical test. Arch. Neurol. **35**(6), 364–367 (1978)
32. Money, J., Alexander, D., Walker, H.T.: A standardized road-map test of direction sense: Manual. Johns Hopkins Press (1965)
33. Ratcliff, G.: Spatial thought, mental rotation and the right cerebral hemisphere. Neuropsychologia **17**(1), 49–54 (1979)
34. Serino, S., et al.: Assessing the mental frame syncing in the elderly: a virtual reality protocol. Stud. Health Technol. Inform. **199**, 153–157 (2014)

35. Serino, S., et al.: Detecting early egocentric and allocentric impairments deficits in Alzheimer's disease: an experimental study with virtual reality. Front. Aging Neurosci. **7**, 88 (2015)
36. Pietro, C., Silvia, S., Federica, P., Andrea, G., Giuseppe, R.: NeuroVirtual 3D: a multiplatform 3D simulation system for application in psychology and neuro-rehabilitation. In: Ma, M., Jain, L., Anderson, P. (eds.) Virtual Augmented Reality and Serious Games for Healthcare 1, pp. 275–286. Springer, Heidelberg (2014). https://doi.org/10.1007/978-3-642-54816-1_15
37. Colombo, D., et al.: Egocentric and allocentric spatial reference frames in aging: a systematic review. Neurosci. Biobehav. Rev. **80**, 605–621 (2017)
38. Rainville, C., Marchand, N., Passini, R.: Performances of patients with a dementia of the Alzheimer type in the standardized road-map test of direction sense. Neuropsychologia **40** (5), 567–573 (2002)
39. Marková, H., et al.: Perspective taking abilities in amnestic mild cognitive impairment and Alzheimer's disease. Behav. Brain Res. **281**, 229–238 (2015)
40. Pai, M.C., Yang, Y.C.: Impaired translation of spatial representation in young onset Alzheimer's disease patients. Curr. Alzheimer Res. **10**(1), 95–103 (2013)
41. Hegarty, M., Waller, D.: A dissociation between mental rotation and perspective-taking spatial abilities. Intelligence **32**(2), 175–191 (2004)
42. Hort, J., et al.: Spatial navigation deficit in amnestic mild cognitive impairment. Proc. Natl. Acad. Sci. USA **104**(10), 4042–4047 (2007)
43. Laczo, J., et al.: From Morris Water Maze to computer tests in the prediction of Alzheimer's disease. Neurodegener. Dis. **10**(1–4), 153–157 (2012)
44. Laczo, J., et al.: Human analogue of the morris water maze for testing subjects at risk of Alzheimer's disease. Neurodegener. Dis. **7**(1–3), 148–152 (2010)
45. Laczo, J., et al.: Spatial navigation testing discriminates two types of amnestic mild cognitive impairment. Behav. Brain Res. **202**(2), 252–259 (2009)
46. Bellassen, V., et al.: Temporal order memory assessed during spatiotemporal navigation as a behavioral cognitive marker for differential Alzheimer's disease diagnosis. J. Neurosci. **32** (6), 1942–1952 (2012)
47. Morganti, F., Stefanini, S., Riva, G.: From allo-to egocentric spatial ability in early Alzheimer's disease: a study with virtual reality spatial tasks. Cogn. Neurosci. **4**(3–4), 171–180 (2013)
48. Byrne, P., Becker, S., Burgess, N.: Remembering the past and imagining the future: a neural model of spatial memory and imagery. Psychol. Rev. **114**(2), 340 (2007)
49. Burgess, N.: Spatial memory: how egocentric and allocentric combine. Trends Cogn. Sci. **10** (12), 551–557 (2006)

Emerging Technology in Positive Psychology

David B. Yaden[1(✉)], Johannes C. Eichstaedt[1],
and John D. Medaglia[1,2]

[1] University of Pennsylvania, Philadelphia, PA 19104, USA
dyaden@sas.upenn.edu
[2] Drexel University, Philadelphia, PA 19104, USA

Abstract. Technological advances are providing the field of positive psychology with new means with which to potentially enhance well-being. Emerging interventions – such as those from psychopharmacology, noninvasive brain stimulation, apps, big-data computational linguistic analysis of social media, and virtual reality – often diverge in various ways from the primarily cognitive and psychosocial interventions more common in the extant positive psychology literature. This paper describes several of these emerging technologies and considers the effects that they may come to have on the science of well-being, and recommends that positive psychology discourse expand to more fully integrate biopsychosocial aspects of well-being.

Keywords: Positive psychology · Well-being · Enhancement
Psychopharmacology · Noninvasive brain stimulation · Linguistic analysis
Virtual reality · Mental health

1 Introduction

Sociological and historical factors can influence the approaches utilized by a field of research, especially in its early development – and positive psychology is no exception. Despite the adoption of findings and interventions from positive psychology across fields like neuroscience [1] and the humanities [2], positive psychology remains rooted largely in the perspective of cognitive psychology. Martin Seligman, one of the field's founders, was a major figure in the cognitive revolution and is heavily influenced by Aaron Beck, developer of cognitive therapy [3]. While positive psychology has been primarily discussed as a research approach to happiness and well-being that uses rigorous quantitative methods, the theoretical influence of cognitive psychology in positive psychology has been a less explored, yet influential factor in the inception and development of the field.

Accordingly, most positive interventions target cognitive processes, generally through psychosocial interventions [4]. Furthermore, the administration of these interventions typically takes place in face-to-face settings in which a therapist, coach, or trainer conveys information and facilitates evidence-based activities. Examples of this psychosocial, in-person delivery paradigm include University of Pennsylvania programs like Comprehensive Soldier Fitness [5] to prevent mental disorders in soldiers in the US Army, and the Penn Resiliency Program [6] to prevent depressive symptoms in school children. These psychosocial and largely cognitive-based

© ICST Institute for Computer Sciences, Social Informatics and Telecommunications Engineering 2018
P. Cipresso et al. (Eds.): MindCare 2018, LNICST 253, pp. 92–96, 2018.
https://doi.org/10.1007/978-3-030-01093-5_12

intervention programs delivered by in-person trainers have been moderately successful, with reliable well-being enhancements that are relatively small in magnitude.

New technologies, however, are creating novel avenues through which to test and apply well-being interventions. These methods will stretch the field of positive psychology beyond cognitive-based, in-person, psychosocial interventions to include technological advances in biotechnology and information technology. One way to organize these emerging technologies in positive psychology is by using the biopsychoscocial model, widely used in clinical contexts, which acknowledges the influences of biological (e.g. brain mechanisms), psychological (e.g. cognitive processes and emotions), and social (e.g. interpersonal support system) factors on mental health. In this paper, the biopsychosocial model organizes brief reviews of several emerging technologies – psychopharmacology, noninvasive brain stimulation, apps, big-data computational linguistic analysis of social media, and virtual reality – with immediate relevance to research and application in positive psychology. In some cases, these technologies might target cognitive mechanisms directly, whereas others might manipulate biological mechanisms with possible concomitant cognitive changes along with outcome measures of well-being. This paper argues that the field of positive psychology could benefit from more integration of biopsychosocial influences on well-being, especially as several emerging technologies in these categories become more accessible and widely used.

2 Biological

The paucity of mentions of biological research in positive psychology likely springs from superficial distinctions between academic fields, as the cognitive psychology approach tends to focus on non-pharmacological or biological factors. But researchers in the fields of pharmacology and neuroscience have been working on the topic of well-being and, more generally, mental enhancement, for decades [7]. This work is just beginning to become integrated into positive psychology research and discourse.

As for psychopharmacology, there have been several attempts to enhance happiness, usually as an adjunct to the goal of reducing depression and anxiety and often couched in terms of "quality of life." The use of fluoxetine, for example, has at times been described as going beyond meliorating symptoms of depression to enhancing well-being relevant traits, like sociability [8] – though this remains a controversial claim – and it is not clear what specific traits are amenable to alteration from this medication. In any case, psychopharmaceuticals have not been approved by federal regulatory agencies as a means to enhance well-being through prescription and research on such indirect psychological outcomes is still lacking.

While well-being enhancement for chronic-use substances like fluoxetine have generally received only scattered or poor support, the case for certain single-session substances is stronger, though the evidence is still emerging. Research at Johns Hopkins University using the substance psilocybin provides robust support for the possibility of pharmacologically-based well-being enhancement. In one study, Griffiths and colleagues demonstrated that a single session of psilocybin taken in a safe and supportive context reliably increases participants' mood, sense of meaning, and life satisfaction [9], an effect that persists for at least 18 months [10].

In neuroscience, technologies are now available that can leverage decades of neuroimaging findings. Noninvasive brain stimulation technologies can selectively modulate particular patches of cortex imaging studies have shown to be associated with a particular mental function, providing a causal means to test the observed correlations. The most widely used of these technologies, transcranial magnetic stimulation (TMS) and transcranial direct current stimulation (tDCS), can modulate mental functions like learning and mood; as language learning has been shown amenable to enhancement and TMS is becoming part of psychiatric standard of care for treatment resistant depression [11]. While these technologies have not yet been widely tested in terms of their capacity to influence well-being, the identification of several 'hedonic hotspots' [12] throughout the brain provide compelling targets to test, which may eventually provide substantial control over mental processes [13].

3 Psychological

Digital distribution is transforming the delivery of positive interventions. A positive psychology MOOC on Coursera, for example, has already taught many times more students about positive interventions than years of in-person instruction in university settings. The vectors through which psychological findings related to mental health can now be conveyed to the public are unprecedented.

One major way of delivering positive interventions is through apps. Apps like BetterUp, Happify, and Headspace as well as websites like ClearerThinking.org deliver evidence-based well-being interventions to millions of people. In addition to delivery, apps in combination with wearables (or mobile technologies that record data throughout the day) are capable of collecting massive amounts of information [14]. As the interaction with, and integration of, apps and mobile computing devices continues, they will play an increasingly large role in the delivery of positive interventions. Additionally, they will contribute to the awareness of users' fluctuations across well-being relevant domains over seconds, minutes, hours, days, weeks, years, and decades.

Cognitive therapy itself is increasingly being distributed through digital means. The early example of ELIZA, the natural language processing program that allowed users to engage in a therapy-like process [15], has become a reality of clinical research and care. Some studies have examined new fully computerized courses of therapy while others have investigated recently developed computer-assisted courses of cognitive therapy [16]. There is little doubt that well-being interventions will be administered through similar means.

4 Social

Social media is ubiquitous in most western, educated, industrialized, rich, and democratic (WEIRD) countries. Companies like Facebook and Twitter provide massive corpora of language data to study. Viewing and interacting with these social media platforms is a normal part of the day for hundreds of millions of people.

Language data from social media platforms can be used to create highly accurate models of individual psychological characteristics [17]. These characteristics include heart disease [18], demographics like gender [19], personality [20], religious affiliation [21], as well as mental states like self-transcendent experiences (STEs) [22, 23]. Social media posts can also be used to predict mental disorders [24], as well as well-being (e.g. www.WWBP.org).

Initial positive psychology studies on social media tended to focus on the impact of social media use on well-being. This work has evolved to ask more nuanced questions about the surrounding circumstances, individual differences, and manner of interaction with social media [25]. In general, insights from positive psychology about social interactions will likely apply in social media interactions as well: toxic interactions will reduce well-being whereas supportive interactions will increase well-being.

Questions about the impact of social media on well-being will become increasingly important because social media is on the cusp of becoming much more immersive. Virtual reality (VR) is capable of more than inducing intense states of awe [26, 27]; it is also capable of facilitating simulated face-to-face like social interactions through digital avatars [28]. The investment of large social media companies like Facebook in VR companies like Oculus Rift, and the reduction in price of high quality VR headsets, makes immersive virtual social media seem like a likely future reality. However, the well-being dynamics of these virtual social contexts is not yet known with specificity.

5 Conclusion

Positive psychology is at the cusp of moving beyond its cognitive roots to investigate other avenues of studying and enhancing well-being across the biopsychosocial model. Research questions in this domain are no longer of the form of, 'does X technology impact well-being?' but have rather become increasingly complex, now exploring the aims, surrounding circumstances, neurobiology, and ways in which technologies and their applications influence various aspects of well-being. It is imperative that the field of positive psychology integrates technological interventions across biological, psychological, and social influences on well-being. The technologies reviewed here, as well as others, may even go beyond transforming the science of well-being – to transforming the ways in which human beings conceive of and pursue well-being.

References

1. Greene, J., Morrison, I., Seligman, M. (eds.): Positive Neuroscience. Oxford University Press, New York (2016)
2. Tay, L., Pawelski, J.O., Keith, M.G.: The role of the arts and humanities in human flourishing: a conceptual model. J. Posit. Psychol. 13, 1–11 (2017)
3. Seligman, M.E.: Authentic Happiness: Using the New Positive Psychology to Realize Your Potential for Lasting Fulfillment. Simon and Schuster, New York (2004)
4. Rashid, T.: Positive interventions in clinical practice. J. Clin. Psychol. 65(5), 461–466 (2009)
5. Cornum, R., Matthews, M.D., Seligman, M.E.: Comprehensive soldier fitness: building resilience in a challenging institutional context. Am. Psychol. 66(1), 4 (2011)

6. Gillham, J.E., et al.: School-based prevention of depressive symptoms: a randomized controlled study of the effectiveness and specificity of the Penn Resiliency Program. J. Consult. Clin. Psychol. **75**(1), 9 (2007)
7. Farah, M.J.: The unknowns of cognitive enhancement. Science **350**(6259), 379–380 (2015)
8. Kramer, P.D.: Prozac: better than well. Lancet Psychiatry **3**(1), e2–e3 (2016)
9. Griffiths, R.R., Richards, W.A., McCann, U., Jesse, R.: Psilocybin can occasion mystical-type experiences having substantial and sustained personal meaning and spiritual significance. Psychopharmacology **187**(3), 268–283 (2006)
10. Griffiths, R.R., Richards, W.A., Johnson, M.W., McCann, U.D., Jesse, R.: Mystical-type experiences occasioned by psilocybin mediate the attribution of personal meaning and spiritual significance 14 months later. J. Psychopharmacol. **22**(6), 621–632 (2008)
11. Hamilton, R., Messing, S., Chatterjee, A.: Rethinking the thinking cap ethics of neural enhancement using noninvasive brain stimulation. Neurology **76**(2), 187–193 (2011)
12. Berridge, K.C., Kringelbach, M.L.: Neuroscience of affect: brain mechanisms of pleasure and displeasure. Curr. Opin. Neurobiol. **23**(3), 294–303 (2013)
13. Medaglia, J.D., Zurn, P., Sinnott-Armstrong, W., Bassett, D.S.: Mind control as a guide for the mind. Nat. Hum. Behav. **1**(6), s41562-017 (2017)
14. Gaggioli, A., et al.: A mobile data collection platform for mental health research. Pers. Ubiquit. Comput. **17**(2), 241–251 (2013)
15. Weizenbaum, J.: ELIZA—a computer program for the study of natural language communication between man and machine. Commun. ACM **9**(1), 36–45 (1966)
16. Wright, J.H., et al.: Computer-assisted cognitive therapy for depression: maintaining efficacy while reducing therapist time. Am. J. Psychiatry **162**(6), 1158–1164 (2005)
17. Kosinski, M., Stillwell, D., Graepel, T.: Private traits and attributes are predictable from digital records of human behavior. Proc. Natl. Acad. Sci. **110**(15), 5802–5805 (2013)
18. Eichstaedt, J.C., et al.: Psychological language on Twitter predicts county-level heart disease mortality. Psychol. Sci. **26**(2), 159–169 (2015)
19. Park, G., et al.: Women are warmer but no less assertive than men: gender and language on Facebook. PLoS One **11**(5), e0155885 (2016)
20. Schwartz, H.A., et al.: Personality, gender, and age in the language of social media: the open-vocabulary approach. PLoS One **8**(9), e73791 (2013)
21. Yaden, D.B., et al.: The language of religious affiliation: social, emotional, and cognitive differences. Soc. Psychol. Pers. Sci. (2017). https://doi.org/10.1177/1948550617711228
22. Yaden, D.B., et al.: The language of ineffability: linguistic analysis of mystical experiences. Psychol. Relig. Spirit. **8**(3), 244 (2016)
23. Yaden, D.B., Haidt, J., Hood Jr., R.W., Vago, D.R., Newberg, A.B.: The varieties of self-transcendent experience. Rev. Gen. Psychol. **21**(2), 143–160 (2017). https://doi.org/10.1037/gpr0000102
24. Guntuku, S.C., Yaden, D.B., Kern, M.L., Ungar, L.H., Eichstaedt, J.C.: Detecting depression and mental illness on social media: an integrative review. Curr. Opin. Behav. Sci. **18**, 43–49 (2017)
25. Gerson, J., Plagnol, A.C., Corr, P.J.: Subjective well-being and social media use: do personality traits moderate the impact of social comparison on Facebook? Comput. Hum. Behav. **63**, 813–822 (2016)
26. Chirico, A., Yaden, D.B., Riva, G., Gaggioli, A.: The potential of virtual reality for the investigation of awe. Front. Psychol. **7**, 166 (2016)
27. Chirico, A., Cipresso, P., Yaden, D.B., Biassoni, F., Riva, G., Gaggioli, A.: Effectiveness of immersive videos in inducing awe: an experimental study. Sci. Rep. **7**, 1218 (2017)
28. Cipresso, P., Serino, S.: Virtual Reality: Technologies Medical Applications and Challenges. Nova Science Publishers, Inc., Hauppauge (2014)

First Insights into Applying the Game Transfer Phenomena Framework for Positive Means

Angelica B. Ortiz de Gortari[✉]

Psychology and Neuroscience of Cognition Research Unit, University of Liège,
Quartier Agora Place des Orateurs 1 (B33), 4000 Liège, Belgium
angelica@gametransferphenomena.com

Abstract. Gamers have reported that their gaming experiences are pervasive
and manifest even when they are not playing, re-experiencing sensorial perceptions (e.g., seeing images, hearing sounds, voices, tactile sensations), automatic responses toward game-related cues, urges to performed activities as in the
game, etc. This paper proposes applying the Game Transfer Phenomena
(GTP) framework and what has been learned on GTP for: (i) strengthening
interventions using virtual technologies, (ii) developing or enhancing pedagogic
tools for intrusions in mental disorders, and (iii) understanding underlying
symptoms of psychiatric and neurological conditions, including gaming addiction or Internet Gaming Disorder. Can we apply the GTP mechanisms to
develop virtual applications for positive means such as learning skills, modifying interpretation of stimuli, changing dysfunctional habits, etc.? This paper
overviews GTP (e.g., GTP types and characteristics), introduces the GTP
framework, outlines core factors relevant for GTP, GTP mechanisms, and game
contents commonly transferred, and discusses potential applications of GTP.

Keywords: Game Transfer Phenomena · GTP · Video games effects
Virtual reality side-effects · Virtual interventions · Mental disorders
Involuntary phenomena · Mental health

1 Introduction

Playing video games is considered either an enhancer of life experiences, training for
cognitive skills, and a tool for promoting positive means (e.g., rehabilitation, psychopedagogic tool), or as an entertainment activity of concern (e.g., excessive use,
gaming disorder, consumption of controversial contents) [1, 2].

In research on Game Transfer Phenomena (GTP), gamers have reported that game
experiences are pervasive in their life, and manifest even when they are not playing.
Examples include: (i) re-experiencing sensorial perceptions (e.g., seeing images,
hearing sounds, voices, tactile sensations), (ii) automatic responses toward game-
related cues (e.g., objects, environments), (iii) keep replaying the game using real-life

---

Note: The author is beneficiary of the Marie Curie COFUND fellowship, co-funded by the
University of Liège and the European Union.

P. Cipresso et al. (Eds.): MindCare 2018, LNICST 253, pp. 97–106, 2018.
https://doi.org/10.1007/978-3-030-01093-5_13

objects or in real-life sceneries, and (iv) change of behaviors due to video game experiences, etc.

Instead of focusing on the challenges GTP may represent to certain individuals due to the intrusive, spontaneous manner and the circumstances in which some of the GTP are experienced – usually in diurnal contexts when doing automatic activities, including driving – this paper aims to propose the GTP framework, and what has been learned on GTP for (i) strengthening interventions using virtual technologies, (ii) developing or enhancing pedagogic tools for intrusions in mental disorders, and (iii) understanding underlying symptoms of medical conditions (psychological and neurological disorders), including gaming addiction or Internet Gaming Disorder as labelled in the current edition of the DSM (DSM-5) [3].

More specifically, this paper posits the following questions: (i) Can we apply the GTP mechanisms to develop virtual applications for positive means, such as learning skills, modifying interpretation of stimuli, changing dysfunctional habits, etc.? (ii) Can we use the intrusiveness of GTP with neutral or positive content to interfere, distract and reduce unwanted and distressful intrusions such as intrusive thoughts and imagery? The paper is divided into: (i) video game mechanisms, (ii) core factors relevant for GTP, (iii) overview of GTP (e.g., types, characteristics), and (iv) mechanisms of GTP. The paper ends by discussing some of the potential applications of GTP.

1.1 Video Games and Game Mechanisms

Video games are designed as sequences of repetitive events; they have rules, goals, involve progression (e.g., levels), opponents (e.g., competition), and provide scheduled psychological reinforcement and punishment (e.g., rewards, prizes) when goals are accomplished or failed [4]. Moreover, video games pair in-game events with sensory cues with specific meanings of a rewarding or punishing nature which require a response that unchains events [5].

1.2 Core Game Characteristics and In-Game Phenomena Relevant for GTP

GTP appears to be facilitated or enhanced by the practice of repetitive in-game behaviours, prolonged exposure to sensory cues including the repetitive manipulation of game controls, as well as by realism or simulations of physical stimuli, embodiment, and trance states while playing (e.g., immersion in the game) [5–7].

Four core elements related to the video games' structural characteristics and in-game phenomena (e.g., immersion, telepresence) have been proposed as elements that facilitate GTP (see Ortiz de Gortari & Griffiths, 2017, for details on the modalities and types of GTP associated with each of the factors). These are as follows:

Sensory perceptual stimulation – interaction, usually for prolonged periods of time, with repetitive and sometimes stereotypical synthetic sensorial stimuli.

High cognitive load – interactive and demanding activity that requires processing a large variety of sensorial stimuli simultaneously and in a short period of time, involving executive functions, perceptual and motoric skills at play.

Dissociative states – involved in normative dissociative phenomena (i.e., a form of non-pathological dissociation that takes place in recreational activities [8]) such as losing track of time, states of flow, immersion, and sometimes sense of presence and embodiment.

High emotional engagement – rewarding and amusing activity which tends to lead to modification of mood states and physiological responses (e.g., arousal) directly related to in-game events and the gamer's performance in the video game.

2 Overview of GTP

This section includes: (i) GTP definition, types and modalities, (ii) GTP framework, and (iii) main characteristics of GTP (e.g., duration, manifestation, video games and in-game activities associated with GTP).

2.1 Defining GTP and the GTP Framework

GTP is defined as the transfer of experiences from the virtual to the physical world that can manifest as sensorial perceptions, sensations, automatic mental processes, behaviors and actions with video game content.

Altered sensorial perceptions comprise perceptions and/or sensations in all sensorial channels, cross-sensory or multisensory.

Automatic mental processes comprise thoughts, urges and automatic mental actions.

Behaviors and actions comprise a variety of trivial actions to more elaborated behaviors, making distinctions between: (i) *intentional behaviors;* these are deliberately initiated by gamers such as modelling game movements or game characters for amusement, making jokes or using slang to communicate with others, and (ii) *automatic behaviors*, which occur spontaneously and without control under episodic lapses of lack of awareness, usually triggered by game-related cues (Fig. 1).

To explain the interplay of physiological, perceptual, and cognitive mechanisms involved in GTP, a theoretically eclectic approach is used, sustained mainly on socio-cognitive and behavioral theories (e.g., pavlovian conditioning, schema theory, social cognitive theory) based on the premise that our previous experiences influence, at least temporarily and to a variety of degrees, the way we perceive, interpret and respond to the world around us [14].

The GTP framework proposed by de Gortari [14] is not limited to video game contents, game platform, online/offline, excessive playing, dysfunctional or pathological gaming. The GTP framework combines the research fields of video game effects and involuntary phenomena (i.e., sensorial, cognitive or motoric intrusions that arise without premeditation or intention, awareness and control). The GTP framework focuses on examining the relation between structural characteristics of the video games, in-game phenomena (e.g., immersion, trance state, embodiment), and the use of hardware and peripherals, which can influence gamers' sensory perceptions, cognitions and behaviors beyond the game.

In the research on GTP it is very important to make a clear distinction between inner or endogenous experiences from outer or exogenous experiences (e.g., visualizing images vs seeing images in front of the eyes, hearing sounds in the head vs hearing sounds coming from objects associated with the game), as well as to establish the difference between volitional and non-volitional phenomena (e.g., intentional use of slang from a video game vs involuntary verbal outbursts) because it is believed that the psychosocial effects of video games depend on the form and conditions of how GTP manifests [5, 9].

	Altered visual perceptions	Altered auditory perceptions	Altered body perceptions and others	Automatic mental processes	Behaviours & actions
Main Types of GTP per modality	-Mind visualizations/ imagery -Seeing images (closed/open eyes) -Distortions of environments or objects (e.g., shape, color) -Visual misperceptions or confusions of objects.	-Re-plays of music, sounds or voices -Internal monologues -Thoughts voiced out loud -Distortions of sound (e.g., tempo, pitch) -Auditory misperceptions.	-Tactile sensations -Body sensations of self-motion -Involuntary movements of limbs -Uncoordinated movements -Stereotypical body movements -Out of body experiences -Chronoceptive distortions.	- Wanting to use game elements - Still in the mind set of the game: Evaluations based on game logic, irrational expectations, automatic replays of the game, selective attention -Urges to do something as in the game.	-Changes of behaviour -Behaviours influenced by the game -Slips of action/oral slips (e.g., verbal outburst) -Involuntary motoric activations -Activities inspired by the game.
Most prevalent types of GTP	Visualized/seen images w closed eyes.	Re-plays of music from a game.	- Body sensations of self-motion -Tactile sensations.	-Wanting to use game elements in real life -Urges to do something in real life triggered by a game-related cue -Still in the mind set of the game.	Unintentionally sang, shouted or said something with video game contents.

Fig. 1. GTP modalities, types and most prevalent GTP based on three different samples [10–12]

2.2   Characteristics of GTP

Time of manifestation – GTP usually tends to occur hours after or directly after playing, but can also occur within days or later on.

Duration – usually lasts for short periods of time – seconds or minutes – but some gamers have reported effects that last for hours, days and even longer. Some GTP has been reported while playing, although this seems more common with location-based augmented reality games [7]. The duration mainly varies according to the type of modality of GTP. Sensorial experiences (seeing or hearing elements from the game) can last for prolonged periods of time, while thoughts and behaviours usually occur episodically or recurrently.

Circumstances – GTP seems more common in diurnal contexts rather than nocturnal (i.e., lying in bed or trying to sleep), when gamers are doing everyday chores or automatic activities. Thoughts and behaviours usually are triggered by game-related cues or by the resemblance between physical world stimuli and the game, while sensory experiences are less likely to be triggered by associations, but they can also arise from a trigger (e.g., seeing menus during a conversation, seeing a map while searching for an address, seeing power bars above people's heads).

Types of games – GTP has been reported in a large variety of video game genres and platforms, including localisation-based augmented reality games such as *Pokémon Go* [7]. Gamers who reported severe levels of GTP (i.e., experiencing several types of GTP and very frequently) were more likely to report GTP when playing MMORPG, simulation games, adventure games, first-person shooter games, puzzle games, music and dance games and role-playing games, compared to those with moderate or mild levels of GTP.

In-game activities – activities that imply focusing the attention in the game world rather than those related to socialising while playing. These include: i) *exploring* which implies getting immersed in the game activity by discovering, searching, collecting items, paying attention to particular elements and engaging in repetitive activities such as smashing items, approaching corners, etc., and ii) *customising* which requires focusing on appearance, accessorising characters, vehicles and creatively personalising characters by engaging in the repetitive manipulation of game menus.

3   Mechanisms of GTP

Various mechanisms of GTP have been identified which can be useful to have in mind for applying GTP. The most important ones are:

Everyday contexts – GTP is usually experienced in everyday contexts. More common in diurnal contexts rather than nocturnal.

Automatic transfers – GTP is experienced automatically, spontaneously, without awareness and without control.

Preserved contents – the contents from the game are transferred with a high degree of similitude.

Bizarre contents – illogical or bizarre contents that raise awareness.

Triggered by associations – associations between physical stimuli that have been simulated in the game or that resemble those in the game, and video game elements; in general, affordances found in real-life contexts that facilitate associations and allow executions of video game-related activities or actions.

Repeated and recurrent – contents are repeated automatically, sometimes even in an intrusive manner.

Practiced routinely – once game content appears automatically, behaviors can be adopted and become habitual, sometimes in a playful way. Some practice them even in a compulsive manner.

Modification of processes – at least temporary changes in cognition (e.g., interpretations of physical stimuli associated with the virtual experience), perceptions (e.g., perceiving physical stimuli with different characteristics – color, shape, velocity) and behavior (e.g., change of behavior toward game-related cues-approach, avoid, etc.) (Fig. 2).

	Altered visual perceptions	Altered auditory perceptions	Altered body perceptions	Automatic mental processes	Behaviours & actions
Examples of game elements transferred	Feedback features/Game accessories: maps, Power bars, HUD, menus, Cross hairs Special visual effects (change in color, slow motion, etc.) Stereotypical images.	Background music Percussive, binaural sounds Sounds of lasers, bullets, explosions Beeps, rings, coins steps, vehicles Voices, screams Whispers.	Slow motion, high velocity, feeling as if flying, bouncing, etc. Embodying big/small characters Pushing buttons, haptic control.	Game strategies Game mechanisms Activities: Tracking objects, searching, exploring, climbing, jumping, running, hiding, driving, arranging, counting steps.	Mimicking body positions, walking style, using game slang Activities: picking, hiding, exploring, jumping, walking, running, hunting, flying.
GTP examples	"I get different answering options as a picture in my head from Dragon Age. My sister insulted me, and I thought "What am I going to answer?" Right back at you!" "I see it as options in my head... the game triggered it ... I feel organized" "Every time I talk to someone, the 'Mass Effect' conversation wheel comes up at the bottom of my vision"	"Every time someone welcomes me, no matter the phrase I hear 'Wind' from Castlevania: Portrait of Ruin in my head saying 'you are back'" "After years of playing Outrun whenever I drive under a sign on the road, I hear in my head 'CHECKPOINT'!"	"Our subway system often announces stops and service, and I swear it feels as if I'm Gordon Freeman going into work every morning" "'feel' the constant movement of an arena fight...I had done the whole damn arena list before bed. I can liken this to feeling the waves at the beach after you get home"	"Overwhelming urge to shoot at CCTV cameras, or at least stay out of their line of sight" "Once I stayed up all night to play Lemmings. The next day, when I was trying to read, I kept trying to figure out how to get the Lemmings across the sentences"	"Need for Speed 2 helped me through a bad slide on ice. When I hit the ice, my brain went into gaming mode. It felt like I was with the controller in my hand...I ended up off the slide" "I haven't played a Zelda game for 2 years...I was looking in the drawers a game. When I found it without even realising I sang the open chest theme"

Fig. 2. Examples of video game elements transferred in each modality and GTP experiences.

4   Applications and Potential Applications of GTP

GTP offers a broad **frame for assessing the effects derived from the use of virtual technologies that:** (i) takes into account the interplay between physiological, psychological and social aspects, (ii) is not limited to a video game genre, platform, online/offline or dysfunctional or pathological gaming, and (iii) considers digital contents and their structural characteristics, the interaction with hardware (e.g., keyboard) and in-game phenomena (e.g., immersion, embodiment, telepresence).

GTP can help to identify video game features that provoke discomfort after playing, beyond only looking into psychophysiological side effects (e.g., motion sickness), and potentially reduce risks associated with neural adaptations, particularly when playing using highly immersive technologies, that are believed to strengthen the effects of GTP. A valid and reliable GTP scale with (twenty items) has been developed [13] and a revision is in progress.

Moreover, informing and demystifying GTP appear to be an important contribution to gamers' health, avoiding misinterpretation of normally occurring phenomena which can lead to anxiety, stress and contribute to the development of mental illness, as well as encouraging self-control against performing automatic actions when urges to behave as a response towards game-related cues appear [14].

If the GTP framework [14] is applied with a specific purpose and rigor it may bring some of the following benefits:

4.1 Enhanced Virtual Tools

Identify virtual features (e.g., special sounds, visuals) that cause discomfort, or those that can be included, to: (i) strengthen the effectiveness of interventions using digital tools for therapeutic or pedagogic purposes (e.g., trigger associations, change interpretations of harmful stimuli, change behaviors), or (ii) enhance the engagement with the virtual application.

4.1.1 Take Advantage of Naturally Occurring Phenomena

Naturally occurring mix-ups during the manipulation of virtual technologies can be applied. For example, mobile augmented reality games require the gamer to constantly switch the view between the screen and the real world, which has been found to be associated with mix-ups between the virtual and the real world. More specifically, *Pokémon Go* players have reported looking for Pokémon outside the screen while playing [12].

4.2 Understanding the Underlying Mechanisms of Problematic and Pathological Gaming

Identify and assess factors that contribute to the maintenance and development of symptoms of gaming addiction or Internet Gaming Disorder, and understand further changes in behavior associated with dysfunctional gaming, such as: (i) *selective attention:* focus the attention on particular virtual cues has been found and induced in laboratory settings [15]. GTP also shows this, but in everyday contexts with real-life triggers, where further consequences can be identified (e.g., thought automatization, change of behavior, or even sensorial intrusions when gamers see images or hear sounds guided by top-down processing or by sensory cortex activations triggered by game-related cues [16]), (ii) *identify thought mechanisms* associated with the game (e.g., content, irrationality), (iii) *neural adaptations and over-sensitization to stimuli* that may be related with the activation of dopaminergic neurotransmissions associated with game elements and rewarding virtual experiences.

Other potential applications of assessing GTP in video games and the general use of virtual technologies include:

4.3 Clinical-Related Contexts

Various clinical applications can be exploited including mimicking symptoms of medical conditions for psychopedagogic or research purposes. This is because phenomenological similarities (e.g., circumstances of manifestation, type of phenomena) have been observed between GTP and symptoms of mental disorders (e.g., schizophrenia, Hallucinogen Persistent Perceptual disorder, alcohol withdrawal, sleep disorders) [17].

4.3.1 Psychopedagogic Tool
This can be used in diverse ways: (i) **psychopedagogic tool with patients:** it can help to explain their symptoms to patients outside the frame of pathology, learning about the commonality of intrusions in the non-clinical population; and learning about the mechanisms of involuntary phenomena and perhaps encourage strategies to confront, reduce or tolerate them, (ii) **promote empathy towards mental illness in the general population:** simulation of hallucinations via voice simulation tapes [18] or virtual reality simulation [19] have been used to reduce stigma among the non-clinical population. GTP experiences can be used for explaining that involuntary phenomena can also be experienced by common activities such as playing video games, explain the GTP mechanisms, evolution from intrusions to change on behavior, etc. To this end, a collection of over 60 cartoons based on gamers' experiences has been created to explain GTP to the general public[1].

4.3.2 Investigate Symptoms of Medical Conditions
Investigate individuals who are highly prone to certain GTP types for understanding symptoms and underlying mechanisms of medical conditions. Moreover, GTP can be used for investigating symptoms such as *overreaction toward stimuli* – social anxiety disorders (PTSD, phobias); *hallucinations, delusions* – schizophrenia; *perseverative mental states, sensory sensibility* – autism; *nocturnal involuntary movements, eidetic images, imagery, hypnagogic* – sleep disorders.

4.3.3 A Tool for Evaluating Therapeutic Interventions Using Video Games/VR
Evaluate the effects of the intervention in the everyday life of the patient for: (i) avoiding unwanted effects (e.g., intrusive thoughts, hallucinations) derived from interventions using virtual technologies, (ii) identifying factors that reduce or interfere in the treatment or reduce its efficacy (e.g., harmful automatic associations between virtual elements and real-life elements), (iii) identifying which virtual elements are transferred and how they are transferred into real-life settings for potentially using them to enhance the treatment.

4.4 Enhanced Interventions

Playing video games, mainly *Tetris* (a tile puzzle game), has been used for taxing the visuospatial resources required for the formation of flashbacks in PTSD or cravings in addictions in lab environments [20] and in real-life settings [21, 22] with a degree of success. Ortiz de Gortari and Griffiths have argued that the intrusiveness of GTP (e.g.,

[1] http://gametransferphenomena.com/resources/cartoons/.

recurrent images, thoughts about the game) may play a role or can be used to strengthen interventions using video games for reducing, interfering or substituting the unwanted and distressful intrusions with neutral contents [23].

4.5 Predictive Tool for Future Development of Medical Conditions

Perhaps it could be useful to identify individual characteristics associated with the proneness to develop future medical conditions or cognitive impairment, e.g., identify individuals in prodromal phases to develop psychotic illness. For instance, research has found that Parkinson patients without a history of hallucinations experienced them during a virtual intervention, and years later only this group reported development of hallucinations [24].

5 Conclusion

Research on GTP has from a novel perspective demonstrated how playing video games can lead to at least temporary changes in cognition, sensorial perception and behaviors in everyday contexts, especially how associations between physical stimuli (e.g., objects, environments) and video game elements and experiences are automatically established after playing games.

The author believes that if GTP mechanisms are applied with specific purposes and rigor it is possible to take advantage of GTP, e.g., modifying interpretation of real-life stimuli associated with distress, interfere or replacing distressful thoughts and unwanted sensorial material such as imagery, voices, etc. The applications of GTP remain to be tested and the GTP framework should be applied carefully, having in mind that some gamers (at least 20%) have reported distress or dysfunction at some point due to GTP [10], and also that transfer of effects requires a certain amount of time to settle down (i.e., frequent gaming and prolonged gaming sessions). More research on GTP is needed to better understand the mechanisms and characteristics of GTP that can potentially be used either to enhance the effectiveness of virtual tools/virtual experiences, or for developing interventions based on naturally and commonly occurring involuntary phenomena with digital content that have a long-term effect.

References

1. Griffiths, M.D., Kuss, D.J., de Gortari, A.B.O.: Videogames as therapy: an updated selective review of the medical and psychological literature. Int. J. Priv. Health Inf. Manag. **5**, 71–96 (2017)
2. Greitemeyer, T.: Intense acts of violence during video game play make daily life aggression appear innocuous: a new mechanism why violent video games increase aggression. J. Exp. Soc. Psychol. **50**, 52–56 (2014)
3. APA: Diagnostic and Statistical Manual of Mental Disorders (DSM-5), Washington DC (2013)
4. Dill, K.E., Dill, J.C.: Video game violence: a review of the empirical literature. Aggress. Violent Behav. **3**, 407–428 (1999)

5. de Gortari, A.B.O., Griffiths, M.D.: Automatic mental processes, automatic actions and behaviours in Game Transfer Phenomena: an empirical self-report study using online forum data. Int. J. Mental. Health Addict. **12**, 432–452 (2014)
6. Shapiro, S., Rotter, M.: Graphic depictions: portrayals of mental illness in video games. J. Forensic Sci. **61**, 1592–1595 (2016)
7. de Gortari, A.B.O.: Empirical study on Game Transfer Phenomena in a location-based augmented reality game. Telemat. Inform. (in press)
8. Butler, L.D.: Normative dissociation. Psychiatr. Clin. North Am. **29**, 45–62 (2006)
9. de Gortari, A.B.O., Griffiths, M.D.: Altered visual perception in Game Transfer Phenomena: an empirical self-report study. Int. J. Hum.-Comput. Interact. **30**, 95–105 (2014)
10. de Gortari, A.B.O., Griffiths, M.D.: Prevalence and characteristics of Game Transfer Phenomena: a descriptive survey study. Int. J. Hum.-Comput. Interact. **32**, 470–480 (2016)
11. Dindar, M., de Gortari, A.B.O.: Turkish validation of the Game Transfer Phenomena Scale (GTPS): measuring altered perceptions, automatic mental processes and actions and behaviours associated with playing video games. Telemat. Inform. **34**, 1802–1813 (2017)
12. de Gortari, A.B.O.: Empirical study on Game Transfer Phenomena in a localization-based augmented reality game. Telemat. Inform. (in press). https://doi.org/10.1016/j.tele.2017.12.015
13. de Gortari, A.B.O., Pontes, H., Griffiths, M.D.: The Game Transfer Phenomena Scale: an instrument for investigating the non-volitional effects of video game playing. Cyberpsychology Behav. Soc. Netw. **18**, 588–594 (2015)
14. de Gortari, A.B.O.: The Game Transfer Phenomena framework: investigating altered perceptions, automatic mental processes and behaviors induced by virtual immersion. Ann. Rev. Cybertherapy Telemed. **9**, 9–15 (2016)
15. Boot, W.R., Kramer, A.F., Simons, D.J., Fabiani, M., Gratton, G.: The effects of video game playing on attention, memory, and executive control. Acta Psychol. **129**, 387–398 (2008)
16. de Gortari, A.B.O., Griffiths, M.D.: Beyond the boundaries of the game: the interplay between in-game phenomena, structural characteristics of video games, and game transfer phenomena A2 - Gackenbach, Jayne. In: Bown, J. (ed.) Boundaries of Self and Reality Online, pp. 97–121. Academic Press, San Diego (2017)
17. de Gortari, A.B.O., Larøi, F., Lerner, A.: Can game transfer phenomena contribute to the understanding of the psychophysiological mechanisms of gaming disorder? A comparison of visual intrusions induced by videogames and mental disorders. In: 4th International Conference on Behavioural Addictions, pp. 9–10 (2012). J. Behav. Add.
18. Ando, S., Clement, S., Barley, E.A., Thornicroft, G.: The simulation of hallucinations to reduce the stigma of schizophrenia: a systematic review. Schizophr. Res. **133**, 8–16 (2011)
19. Penn, D.L., Ivory, J.D., Judge, A.: The virtual doppelganger: effects of a virtual reality simulator on perceptions of schizophrenia. J. Nerv. Mental Dis. **198**, 437–443 (2010)
20. Holmes, E.A., James, E.L., Coode-Bate, T., Deeprose, C.: Can playing the computer game "Tetris" reduce the build-up of flashbacks for trauma? A proposal from cognitive science. PLoS ONE **4**, e4153 (2009)
21. Iyadurai, L., et al.: Preventing intrusive memories after trauma via a brief intervention involving Tetris computer game play in the emergency department: a proof-of-concept randomized controlled trial. Mol. Psychiatry **23**, 674–682 (2018)
22. Skorka-Brown, J., Andrade, J., Whalley, B., May, J.: Playing Tetris decreases drug and other cravings in real world settings. Addict. Behav. **51**, 165–170 (2015)
23. de Gortari, A.B.O., Griffiths, M.D.: Commentary: Playing the computer game tetris prior to viewing traumatic film material and subsequent intrusive memories: examining proactive interference. Front. Psychol. **7**, 260 (2016)
24. Albani, G., Pedroli, E., Cipresso, P., et al.: Visual hallucinations as incidental negative effects of virtual reality on Parkinson's disease patients: a link with neurodegeneration? Parkinson's Dis. **2015**, 6 p. (2015). Article ID 194629. https://doi.org/10.1155/2015/194629

Engaging Elderly Breast Cancer Patients Through an e-health Intervention: A Case Series Study

Daniela Villani[1(⊠)], Chiara Cognetta[2], Davide Toniolo[2],
Francesco Scanzi[3], and Giuseppe Riva[1,4]

[1] Department of Psychology, Università Cattolica del Sacro Cuore, Milan, Italy
{daniela.villani,giuseppe.riva}@unicatt.it
[2] Department of Medical Oncology, "G.Salvini" ASST Rodhense, Milan, Italy
cognettachiara@gmail.com, toniolodoc@gmail.com
[3] U.O. Oncologia Medica, Ospedale S. Giuseppe- Multimedica, Milan, Italy
francesco.scanzi@multimedica.it
[4] Applied Technology for Neuro-Psychology Lab,
Istituto Auxologico Italiano, Milan, Italy

Abstract. The aging population increases the number of new diagnoses of breast cancer and women of all ages experience psychological stress for possible treatment related side effects. To prepare elderly women diagnosed with breast cancer to face the imminent chemotherapy we developed an e-health intervention based on the Stress Inoculation Training (SIT) protocol, lasting two weeks. The online intervention includes 10 sessions to see once a day. The research design is a controlled trial comparing an experimental group, following the online intervention in addition to traditional treatment provided by the hospital, and a control group without treatment. The aim of this contribution is to explore the level of engagement of eight patients through a case series study. Furthermore, the acceptance of the online intervention by elderly patients in terms of perceived pleasantness, usefulness and easiness is assessed. Data show that patients remain in a stable position (mainly ranging from the arousal and the adhesion phases) within the engagement process after two weeks. Furthermore, patients of the experimental group report a good level of acceptance of the e-health intervention. Thus, preliminary results suggest that the e-health intervention is well accepted by elderly patients and that it addresses patients' need of knowing the imminent treatment experience and of understanding how to deal with it.

Keywords: e-health · Patient engagement · Breast cancer · Acceptance
Online intervention

1 Introduction

Breast cancer is the most common cancer in women in the world and its incidence still increases, even if at a slower rate, in women aged over 50 years until age of 80 years [1]. Actually the incidence of breast cancer represents a critical health concern in the growing ageing population and requires specific evidence-based recommendations

© ICST Institute for Computer Sciences, Social Informatics and Telecommunications Engineering 2018
P. Cipresso et al. (Eds.): MindCare 2018, LNICST 253, pp. 107–114, 2018.
https://doi.org/10.1007/978-3-030-01093-5_14

[2, 3]. Among several treatment options, chemotherapy treatment is experienced as distressing and traumatizing for women with different ages [4]. In particular, hair loss, nausea and fatigue are frequently ranked among the first three important side effects for breast cancer patients [5, 6]. Some studies suggest that the possibility of anticipating side effects and developing coping strategies can make the experience less stressful [7, 8].

Therefore, sustaining the engagement of breast cancer patients at different ages represents an important aim [9]. Specifically, according to the model proposed by Graffigna and colleagues, patient engagement can be defined as a processual multi-level experience resulting from conjoint cognitive, emotional and conative orientation of individuals towards their health management and it is composed of four incremental and evolutionary phases [10, 11]. In the *blackout phase*, patients fall into an initial state of emotional, behavioural and cognitive blackout determined by a critical event (the diagnosis or the communication of the upcoming chemotherapy) that appears unexpected and out of their control. The period before the initation of adjuvant chemotherapy may overlap with the second phase of the engagement process (*arousal phase*). Breast cancer patient are hyper attentive for all symptoms their bodies produce and these symptoms can cause patients anxiety. Thanks to the increase of knowledge about the treatment and its related side effects and the acquisition of coping strategies, patients start to feel sufficiently confident in their own emotional strength (*adhesion phase*). At the end of the process, usually after having completed the treatment, breast cancer patients have a chance to recapture a positive life planning oriented to the future (*eudaimonic project phase*).

e-health interventions are recognized to have a tremendous potential to promote patient engagement [12], as they allow to develop integrated, sustainable and patient-centered services, to promote and enhance health and to augment the efficacy and efficiency of the process of healthcare [13]. A recent analysis of the literature identified different e-health approaches aiming to sustain breast cancer women engagement [14]. One is the narrative approach, that typically includes the use of personal websites to help patients to express their emotions and enhance their emotional well-being [15]. A second is the support group approach, that usually aims to enhance social support through online peer support interventions. Recently older women reported that they receive several benefits from using online support groups especially about the feeling of being in control of their health [16]. A third approach proposes online training aimed to help patients to manage their affective state and acquire coping strategies. With this aim, recently Villani and colleagues [17] developed a two weeks e-health intervention based on Meichenbaum's Stress Inoculation Training (SIT) [18] protocol for helping elderly women undergoing chemotherapy to cope with impeding treatment side effects. The protocol was composed by three phases coherent with the general SIT objectives: (1) increasing knowledge about the stress process, (2) developing self-regulation skills and (3) helping individual to use the acquired coping skills in real contexts. The clinical rationale behind this approach is to "inoculate" the stressor in patient's experience, in combination with the acquisition of effective coping skills, so that patients could be prepared when they will encounter the critical experience of chemotherapy.

According to a recent systematic review [19], cyberSIT appears to be a promising clinical approach, and Villani and colleagues tested its effectiveness on anxiety reduction and coping skills improvement with a sample of oncology nurses [20]. Overall, the SIT protocol activates the three components of patient engagement: cognitive (by increasing what the patient knows, understands and how she makes sense of the disease and its treatments), emotional (by developing awareness about patient's own emotional reactions and learning adaptive emotion regulation skills) and behavioral (by stimulating specific activities to face the disease and the treatments, such as coping with hair loss).

As investigated by Fogel and colleagues [21], variables as age, length of time since diagnosis, and breast cancer stage are unrelated to Internet use. Furthermore, an increasing number of women patients of any age are accessing health information on the Internet [22]. Specifically, the acceptance of e-health technologies represents a critical factor influencing their effective use and thus fostering the active role of patients in their healthcare. One of the most influential models in explaining user acceptance of information technology is the Technology Acceptance Model (TAM) [23] that hypothesizes two fundamental factors affecting people's attitudes toward IT and influencing at its turn the intention to use and the actual usage of technologies: *perceived usefulness* and *perceived ease of use*. Furthermore, as analyzed by other studies (Villani et al., in press), the positive affective attitude (*pleasantness*) towards technologies represents an addictional dimension of technology acceptance.

The aim of this contribution is to explore the level of engagement of eight elderly breast cancer patients through a case series study. Furthermore, we are interested in assessing the acceptance of the e-health intervention in terms of perceived pleasantness, usefulness and easiness of the proposed experiences.

2 Method

2.1 Participants

The intervention was proposed to all breast cancer patients which was offered chemotherapy in two hospitals of Milan. Inclusion criteria were: age >55 years old; diagnosis of breast cancer radically operated; negative staging for distant metastases; and suitability for adjuvant chemotherapy with anthracyclines and taxanes. All patients decided voluntarily to participate and they gave written informed consent before being enrolled in the study. Patients were allowed to withdraw from the study whenever they wanted. Ethic approval was attained from the Ethics Committee of Department of Psychology of the Università Cattolica del Sacro Cuore, Milan (Italy).

Eight breast cancer patients were included in the study (Table 1). Patients 1, 2, 3 and 4 followed the e-health intervention for two weeks; patients 5, 6, 7 and 8 were included in the control group without intervention and received the usual care for two weeks. The usual care during the two weeks before chemotherapy consists of waiting for the imminent treatment.

Table 1. Characteristics of patients

	e-health group				Control Group			
	P1	P2	P3	P4	P5	P6	P7	P8
Age	60	58	70	58	66	65	55	58
Education level	High school	Junior high school	M.S. Degree	Elementary school	Elementary school	Junior high school	Junior high school	High school
Marital status	Married	Divorced	Married	Never Married	Married	Married	Married	Married
Occupational status	Employed	Employed	Retired	Housewife	Housewife	Housewife	Employed	Freelance worker

Demographic characteristics included age education level (elementary school, junior high school, high school, M.S. degree); marital status (married, never married, widowed, cohabitation, or divorced) and occupational status (housewife, employed, freelance worker, or retired).

2.2   e-health Intervention

The e-health intervention based on Meichenbaum's SIT intervention [18] aimed to facilitate anticipatory coping of elderly women undergoing chemotherapy. The e-health intervention *Con il seno di poi* (Table 2) has been delivered online (www. conilsenodipoi.it). During the first meeting with the psychologist, patients were invited to reflect on the nature of the psychological stress due to disease and upcoming treatment in order to achieve a greater consciousness about its main components (conceptualization phase of the SIT protocol). In this session patients experienced a live-video simulation of a chemotherapy session that they will receive within a few weeks. Furthermore, they received the access to the online intervention for a period of 14 days. During that time, the psychologist's personal contact has been provided.

2.3   Measures

Patient Health Engagement Scale (PHE-S) developed by Graffigna and colleagues [26] was used to measure patient engagement. Patients fulfilled in the scale with the psychologist before the intervention and at the end of the intervention, after two weeks. The scale consists of 5 ordinal items and is based on a conceptual model of patient engagement (PHE- model), which features four positions along a continuum of engagement (i.e., blackout; arousal; adhesion; eudaimonic project).

Patients' acceptance of e-health intervention has been assessed through ad hoc questions aimed to assess the live-video interviews with women who have gone through breast cancer experience (pleasantness and usefulness) and meditation experiences (pleasantness, usefulness, and easiness). Each aspect has been assessed through one ad hoc item with 7 response options on a Likert scale. Patients answered these ad hoc question online after each session. The mean value among the ten online sessions has been calculated for each dimension and for each patient.

Table 2. e-health intervention *Con il seno di poi*

SIT phase	Content of the experience
Skills acquisition and rehearsal phase (online sessions 1–7)	The multimedia experience includes seven 25 min sessions to see once a day. Each session includes two parts. In the first one, patients can watch live-video interviews with women who have gone through breast cancer experience, with particular attention to their expectations and emotions, to chemotherapy side effects and to strategies to cope with changes. In the second part, a relaxation and meditation experience is proposed. Specifically, a natural relaxing video is integrated with narrative audio. Exercises are based on muscle progressive relaxation (focusing on legs, arms, abdome, shoulders, face, front, etc.) [24] and breathing. More, the narrative includes Mindfulness inspired strategies [25], such as thought contemplation and detached mindfulness, useful to be aware of one's thoughts and emotions associated with them, and to look at the problem from a different perspective
Application and follow - through phase (sessions 8–10)	The multimedia experience includes three 25 min sessions to see once a day. Also in this case, each session includes two parts. First, video-live of breast cancer patients' interviews currently undergoing chemotherapy treatments - both with and without wigs - are presented. In this way women directly deal with changes due to illness, chemotherapy and related side effects. In addition, suggestions proposed by other patients offer the chance of anticipate possible solutions to problems they will have to cope with. Second, supported by a natural relaxing video integrated with narrative audio, women are encouraged to apply relaxation and meditation strategies acquired in the previous phase sessions

3 Results

3.1 Patients' Engagement

According to the PHE-S, patients can be positioned along a continuum of engagement ranging from the *blackout* phase to the *eudaimonic project* phase. As shown in Table 3, patients maintain a stable position in the *arousal* or *adhesion* phases after two weeks (the duration of the intervention). Specifically, this happens for patients 3 and 4 of the e-health intervention group, while patient 2 evolves from the *blackout* phase to the *arousal* phase and patient 1 comes from the *adhesion* phase back to the *arousal* phase. Patients of the control group maintain a stable position after two weeks, except for patient 6 which evolves from the *blackout* phase to the *arousal* phase.

Table 3. Patients' engagement positions

	e-health group				Control group			
	P1	P2	P3	P4	P5	P6	P7	P8
Baseline	Adhesion	Blackout	Adhesion	Arousal	Arousal	Blackout	Adhesion	Adhesion
After two weeks	Arousal	Arousal	Adhesion	Arousal	Arousal	Arousal	Adhesion	Adhesion

3.2 Patients' Acceptance of the e-health Intervention

The level of patients' acceptance of the e-health intervention (Table 4) comprises patients' evaluation of the two experiences proposed within each online session (interview and meditation) in term of pleasantness, usefulness and easiness. Each dimension is described along a continuum ranging from 1 ("Not at all") to 7 ("Extremely"). Patients 1 and patient 4 reported higher scores of acceptance than patients 2 and 3. In general, all acceptance considered dimensions reached a positive evaluation.

Table 4. Acceptance of e-health intervention

	P1	P2	P3	P4	Total M (SD)
Live-video interview pleasantness	6.67	4.92	4.90	6.25	5.69 (.91)
Live-video interview usefulness	6.84	5.20	4.90	6.18	5.78 (.89)
Meditation pleasantness	6.34	4.67	5.20	6.18	5.60 (.80)
Meditation usefulness	6.59	5.00	4.90	6.18	5.67 (.85)
Meditation easiness	6.84	6.58	6.45	6.07	6.49 (.32)

4 Discussion

This contribution provides the first examination of the effects of an e-health intervention for elderly women undergoing chemotherapy on their engagement and intervention acceptance. Eight women completed the trial, and these primary results are promising.

On the one hand, patients of both groups maintained a stable position about health engagement (mainly ranging from the arousal and the adhesion phases) after two weeks. Even if health engagement appears similar in the two groups, we have to consider that two weeks are a short time to promote patients' engagement. The research is still ongoing and future analyses should include a follow-up evaluation in order to investigate whether the effects of the e-health intervention on patient engagement can be enhanced over time. Furthermore, future research efforts should investigate and define how to design oncology processes of care including e-health intervention that support patient engagement in meaningful ways [27].

On the other hand, patients of the experimental group reported a good level of acceptance of the e-health intervention. Live-video interviews were assessed as useful and pleasant. Meditation experiences were primarily assessed as very easy to be applied and also useful and pleasant. This result appears coherent with other studies showing that brief mindfulness meditation protocols can be successfully integrated in self-help interventions supported by new technologies and mobile apps [28–30].

This study has some limitations that should be highlighted. First, findings are preliminary and results coming from the case series analysis cannot be generalized to a wider population. Data collection from a wider sample is needed to allow statistical comparisons between groups and to confirm the acceptance of the intervention.

Nevertheless, preliminary results suggest that the proposed e-health intervention represents a promising and acceptable approach to prepare elderly women to cope with the stressful experience of chemotherapy.

Acknowledgments. This study has been supported by Catholic University of Sacred Heart of Milan (D3.2 Tecnologia Positiva e Healthy Aging - Positive Technology and Healthy Aging, 2014).

References

1. DeSantis, C., Siegel, R., Bandi, P., Jemal, A.: Breast cancer statistics. CA Cancer J. Clin. **61**(6), 408–418 (2011)
2. Petrakis, I.E., Paraskakis, S.: Breast cancer in the elderly. Arch. Gerontol. Geriatr. **50**(2), 179–184 (2010)
3. Biganzoli, L., et al.: Management of elderly patients with breast cancer: updated recommendations of the International Society of Geriatric Oncology (SIOG) and European Society of Breast Cancer Specialists (EUSOMA). Lancet Oncol. **13**(4), e148–e160 (2012)
4. Browall, M., Gaston-Johansson, F., Danielson, E.: Post-menopausal women with breast cancer: their experiences of the chemotherapy treatment period. Cancer Nurs. **29**(1), 34–42 (2006)
5. Carelle, N., Piotto, E., Bellanger, A., Germanaud, J., Thuillier, A., Khayat, D.: Changing patient perceptions of the side effects of cancer chemotherapy. Cancer **95**(1), 155–163 (2002)
6. Lindop, E., Cannon, S.: Experiences of women with a diagnosis of breast cancer: a clinical pathway approach. Eur. J. Oncol. Nurs. **5**, 91–99 (2001)
7. Frith, H., Harcourt, D., Fussell, A.: Anticipating an altered appearance: women undergoing chemotherapy treatment for breast cancer. Eur. J. Oncol. Nurs. **11**(5), 385–391 (2007)
8. Golant, M., Altman, T., Martin, C.: Managing cancer side effects to improve quality of life: a cancer psychoeducation program. Cancer Nurs. **26**, 37–44 (2003)
9. Graffigna, G., Barello, S., Riva, G., Bosio, A.C.: Patient engagement: the key to redesign the exchange between the demand and supply for healthcare in the era of active ageing. Stud. Health. Technol. Inform. **203**, 85–95 (2014). https://doi.org/10.3233/978-1-61499-425-1-85
10. Graffigna, G., Barello, S., Riva, G.: How to make health information technology effective: the challenge of patient engagement. Arch. Phys. Med. Rehabil. **94**, 2034–2035 (2013). https://doi.org/10.1016/j.apmr.2013.04.024
11. Graffigna, G., Barello, S., Riva, G.: Technologies for patient engagement (Millwood). Health. Aff. **32**, 1172 (2013). https://doi.org/10.1377/hlthaff.2013.0279
12. Barello, S., et al.: e-health for patient engagement: a systematic review. Front. Psychol. **6**, 1–13 (2016). https://doi.org/10.3389/fpsyg.2015.02013
13. Eysenbach, G.: What is e-health? J. Med. Internet. Res. **3**, 20 (2001). https://doi.org/10.2196/jmir.3.2.e20
14. Villani, D., Cognetta, C., Toniolo, D., Scanzi, F., Riva, G.: Engaging elderly breast cancer patients: the potential of e-health interventions. Front. Psychol. **7**, 1825 (2016). https://doi.org/10.3389/fpsyg.2016.01825
15. Harris, L.N., Cleary, E.H., Stanton, A.L.: Project connect online: user and visitor experiences of an internet-based intervention for women with breast cancer. Psycho-Oncol. **24**(9), 1145–1151 (2015)

16. Seçkin, G.: I am proud and hopeful: age-based comparisons in positive coping affect among women who use online peer-support. J. Psychosoc. Oncol. **29**(5), 573–591 (2011)
17. Villani, D., Cognetta, C., Toniolo, D., Riva, G.: Helping women with breast cancer to cope with hair loss: an e-SIT Protocol. Commun. Comput. Inf. Sci. (2016). https://doi.org/10.1007/978-3-319-32270-4_1
18. Meichenbaum, D.: Stress Inoculation Training. Pergamon Press, New York (1985)
19. Serino, S., Triberti, S., Villani, D., Cipresso, P., Gaggioli, A., Riva, G.: Toward a validation of cyber-interventions for stress disorders based on stress inoculation training: a systematic review. Virtual Real. **18**(1), 73–87 (2014)
20. Villani, D., Grassi, A., Cognetta, C., Toniolo, D., Cipresso, P., Riva, G.: Self-help stress management training through mobile phones: an experience with oncology nurses. Psychol. Serv. **10**(3), 315–322 (2013)
21. Fogel, J., Albert, S.M., Schnabel, F., Ditkoff, B.A., Neugut, A.I.: Use of the Internet by women with breast cancer. J. Med. Internet Res. **4**(2), e9 (2002). https://doi.org/10.2196/jmir.4.2.e9
22. Davis, F.: Perceived usefulness, perceived ease of use, and user acceptance of information technology. MIS Q. **13**(3), 319–340 (1989)
23. Villani, A., et al.: Students' acceptance of tablet PCs in Italian high schools: profiles and differences. Br. J. Educ. Technol. **49**(3), 533–544 (2018). https://doi.org/10.1111/bjet.12591
24. Jacobson, E.: Progressive Relaxation. University of Chicago Press, Chicago (1938)
25. Kabat-Zinn, J.: Mindfulness-based interventions in context: past, present, and future. Clin. Psychol. Sci. Pract. **10**(2), 144–156 (2003)
26. Graffigna, G., Barello, S., Bonanomi, A., Lozza, E.: Measuring patient engagement: development and psychometric properties of the Patient Health Engagement (PHE) Scale. Front. Psychol. **6**, 274 (2015). https://doi.org/10.3389/fpsyg.2015.00274
27. Bosworth, H.B., Pini, T.M., Walters, C.B., Sih-Meynier, R.: The future of patient engagement in the oncology setting: how practical patient engagement recommendations and innovative inter-professional education can drive change. J Participat Med. **9**, e7 (2017)
28. Carissoli, C., Villani, D., Riva, G.: Does a meditation protocol supported by a mobile application help people reduce stress? Suggestions from a controlled pragmatic trial. Cyberpsychol. Behav. Soc. Netw. **18**(1), 46–53 (2015)
29. Chittaro, L., Vianello, A.: Evaluation of a mobile mindfulness app distributed through on-line stores: a 4-week study. Int. J. Hum. Comput. Stud. **86**, 63–80 (2016)
30. Ly, K.H., Trüschel, A., Jarl, L., Magnusson, S., Windahl, T., Johansson, R., Andersson, G.: Behavioural activation versus mindfulness-based guided self-help treatment administered through a smartphone application: a randomised controlled trial. BMJ Open **4**, 1 (2014)

Mindful Age and Technology: Promoting Quality of Life in Older Adults with a Tablet/Smartphone App

Francesco Vailati Riboni[1], Benedetta Comazzi[1,4],
Gianluca Castelnuovo[1,2], Enrico Molinari[1,2],
and Francesco Pagnini[1,3(✉)]

[1] Department of Psychology, Universita Cattolica del Sacro Cuore, Milan, Italy
francesco.pagnini@unicatt.it
[2] Istituto Auxologico Italiano, IRCCS, Psychology Research Laboratory,
Verbania, Italy
[3] Department of Psychology, Harvard University, Cambridge, MA, USA
[4] IRCCS Fondazione Don Carlo Gnocchi, Milan, Italy

Abstract. Based on the Langerian definition of mindfulness, we created a smartphone App to promote cognitive flexibility, curiosity, novelty seeking, and creativity in a population of older adults. So far, we have tested it on 68 participants, randomly assigned to the experimental group or to a wait-list control group. Between group comparisons failed to detect a significant effect on quality of life, though qualitative analysis report a positive impact of the App over participants' lives.

Keywords: Mindfulness · Smartphone apps · Older adults · Quality of life

1 Introduction

Ageing and technological innovation are two important topics of current times. As life expectancy has increased, traditional health care systems have faced different challenges in terms of costs-effectiveness as well as high quality services delivery capability [1] New ways to improve older adults' quality of life have been explored, taking advantage of new technological solutions: encouraging different and healthier lifestyles, making non-invasive assessments or delivering distance intervention [2–4]. Recent studies [5] suggest that mindfulness practice may lead to adaptive cognitive schemas' change and emotional self-regulation. Mindfulness can be considered as the simple act of paying attention to novelty, as opposed to being stuck in previous categories and schemas [6]. A mindful outlook is composed by flexibility, openness, curiosity, awareness, and creativity. It plays a key role in the ageing process, both from a psychological and biological perspective [6]. Under these assumptions, a tablet/smartphone application has been developed to promote cognitive flexibility, psychological well-being and an curious attitude to the present moment. The application of advanced technology to psychological and behavioral programs for older adults has been recognized as a promising solution for many issues, including depression, anxiety, and mild cognitive impairment [7].

© ICST Institute for Computer Sciences, Social Informatics and Telecommunications Engineering 2018
P. Cipresso et al. (Eds.): MindCare 2018, LNICST 253, pp. 115–118, 2018.
https://doi.org/10.1007/978-3-030-01093-5_15

2 Methods

The research design of this study is a randomized controlled trial, RCT, aimed to investigate the effect of a mindfulness-based smartphone App on the quality of life of an elderly sample. We were also interested, as secondary aims, to collect information about the effects of the App on psychological well-being, mindfulness disposition, locus of control, depression and anxiety. Participants were randomly assigned to the experimental condition, receiving the App for 14 days, or to a wait-list control group, which received access to the App after three months.

2.1 Assessments

The assessments considered here were conducted at the recruitment (T0, baseline), and after the treatment (T1, post-intervention). The following questionnaire were administered:

- The Psychological General Well-Being Index (PGWBI) was used to evaluate subjective mental health. The 22-item questionnaire is commonly use to generate a self-perceived evaluation of subjects 'psychological well-being expressed by a summary score [8].
- The 14-item version of the Langer Mindfulness Scale (LMS), was used to assess mindfulness. It asses four domains associated with mindful thinking: novelty-seeking, engagement, novelty producing, and flexibility [9].
- The Geriatric Depression Scale (GDS) and the Geriatric Anxiety Inventory (GAI) were used to screen for depression or anxiety within the participants. Both test, specifically designed for the elder population, are largely considered to be able to effectively discriminate between patients with or without depression or anxiety symptoms [10, 11].

Together with the questionnaires, we included a semi-structured interview, which were administered to evaluate subjects' attitude towards technology and related alterations, considered to be influential factors in the acceptance's process and usability of the smartphone application.

2.2 Participants

Participants were recruited with the support of 7 different institutions that provide advance education to older adults. So far, 68 participants where recruited for the protocol from the selected structures. All participants were volunteer.

Inclusion criteria were:

- Age > 65
- Mini-Mental State Examinations, (MMSE; 14) > 18
- No severe neurological or medical condition, according to medical records.

2.3   Intervention

The App was developed with the MIT App Inventor Software (http://appinventor.mit. edu/explore/) and consists of a set of theoretical explanations plus fourteen exercises: half of them linked to logical reasoning while others aimed to share and adopt mindfulness abilities. In the first 7 exercises, participants are cognitively stimulated with simple puzzling tasks, ensuring greater adherence to the protocol due to the ludic engagement experience and easily achievable positive reinforcements resulting from the questions' solution. The other 7 exercises instead require a different approach, stimulating creative and non-conventional solutions, with clear references to everyday situations. Some of the exercises provide audio or video files explaining mindfulness fundamental concept, maintaining an easy and simple language suitable for the specific needs of the users. The entire intervention lasted fourteen days, with one daily exercise/task to be completed. Participants were able to perform all the exercise on their own, wherever they preferred. By completing the first exercise, the App automatically unlocked the next one for the specific next day, allowing users to only complete one task for each day.

3   Results and Discussion

Although this research is still at a preliminary stage, descriptive statistics of data analysis have shown difference between mean score of the groups. In all measured outcomes, participants belonging to the experimental group shown more suitable scores underlining a more adaptive response. Data analyzed in this first stage of the research project, although not statistically relevant, proved to be clinically encouraging (Table 1).

Table 1. Measures collected after the intervention.

Assessment	Intervention group (mean, SD)	Control group (mean, SD)	T-test
PGWBI	88.14 (15.36)	87.9 (11.76)	$t(40) = .056, p = .232$
LMS	1.87 (.07)	1.86 (.08)	$t(40) = .233, p = .861$
GDS	.035 (.29)	.44 (.31)	$t(27) = -.747, p = .817$
GAI	.42 (.429	.53 (.041)	$t(33) = -.781, p = .974$

The qualitative data analysis and codification of the semi-structured interview has highlighted how 45% of the entire sample successfully used the App, while only 7% of the participant declaring not to use it ever. These preliminary data, in line with research hypotheses, show how the elderly population can respond positively to interventions involving different forms of technology, overcoming the stereotype that wants this specific kind of subjects as reluctant to technology. When asked: "Do you believe technology could be useful increasing your wellbeing?", 62% of the subject answered yes, with only 16% of the respondents declaring not to know it clearly. A further analysis of the data collected specifically from the subjects belonging to the experimental condition, found how 66% of the sample have been able to use the smartphone application every day, with only 34% reporting small difficulties with the daily exercise, thus being able to finish the 14-exercise program during the 2 given weeks of the trial.

To the question aimed at understanding how participants felt the applications could have helped them, or what kind of benefits they derived from it, 28% underlined cognitive training, 24% finding alternative and possible solutions to daily problems, 14% highlighted realizing how more points of view could coexist on a single issue and 9% reported mixed benefits, such as memory training or attention improvements.

Since the research protocol is still in progress, further data and specific results analysis will be presented at the conference. This first experimentation of integration between technology and psychology has, however, shown numerous potential, being welcomed by the elderly population and proving to be clinically valid in promoting psychological well-being of the subjects. Future perspectives, therefore, seem to indicate this research line as innovative and extremely important, succeeding in filling a generational gap between psychological demand, technology and clinical practice.

References

1. Stewart, L.: Gerontology: will you still need me, will you still feed me? Nature **514**(7522), S14–S15 (2014)
2. Bercovitz, K., Pagnini, F.: Mindfulness as an opportunity to narrow the grey digital divide. In: Villani, D., Cipresso, P., Gaggioli, A. (eds.) Integrating Technology in Positive Psychology Practice. IGI Global, Hershey 2015
3. Gaggioli, A., et al.: A system for automatic detection of momentary stress in naturalistic settings. Stud. Health Technol. Inf. **181**, 182–186 (2012)
4. Wootton, R.: Twenty years of telemedicine in chronic disease management–an evidence synthesis. J. Telemed. Telecare **18**(4), 211–220 (2012)
5. Langer, E.J., Moldoveanu, M.: The construct of mindfulness. J. Soc. Issues **56**(1), 1–9 (2000)
6. Langer, E.J.: Counterclockwise: Mindful Health and the Power of Possibility. Ballantine Books, New York (2009)
7. Preschl, B., et al.: e-Health interventions for depression, anxiety disorder, dementia, and other disorders in older adults: a review. J. Cyber Ther. Rehabil. **4**(3), 371–385 (2011)
8. Dupuy, H.: The psychological general well-being (PGWB) inventory. In: Wenger, N. (ed.) Assessment of Quality of Life in Clinical Trials of Cardiovascular Therapies, pp. 170–183. Le Jacq Publications, New York (1984)
9. Pirson, M., Langer, E.J., Bodner, T., Zilcha-Mano, S.: The development and validation of the Langer mindfulness scale-enabling a socio-cognitive perspective of mindfulness in organizational contexts. SSRN Electron. J. (2012)
10. Yesavage, J.A., Brink, T.L., Rose, T.L., Lum, D., Huang, V., Adey, M., et al.: Development and validation of a geriatric depression screening scale: a preliminary report. J. Psychiatr. Res. **17**, 37–49 (1983)
11. Pachana, N.A., Byrne, G.J., Siddle, H., Koloski, N., Harley, E., Arnold, E.: Development and validation of the geriatric anxiety inventory. Int. Psychogeriatr. **19**, 103–114 (2007)

Reading Between the Lines: A Computational Bibliometric Analysis on Emotion Regulation

Javier Fernández-Álvarez[1(✉)], Pietro Cipresso[1,2], Desirèe Colombo[3],
Cristina Botella[3], and Giuseppe Riva[1,2]

[1] Department of Psychology of the Catholic University,
Largo Gemelli 1, 20100 Milan, Italy
{javier.fernandezkirszman,giuseppe.riva}@unicatt.it
[2] Applied Technology for Neuro-Psychology Lab at IRCCS Istituto Auxologico
Italiano, Milan, Italy
p.cipresso@auxologico.it
[3] Department of Basic Psychology Clinic and Psychobiology,
Universitat Jaume I, Castellón, Spain
{dcolombo,botella}@uji.es

Abstract. Emotion regulation (ER) is defined as the processes deployed by an individual or group of individuals to explicitly or implicitly influence the experienced emotions in order achieve desirable states or goals. The available literature within this domain has grown exponentially in the last years. Nevertheless, to the best of our knowledge no scientometric analysis has been carried out yet. This kind of analysis allows to grasp how the scientific production within this field is configured, by establishing patterns and connections between the main authorities of the community. In the current analysis, descriptive data of the citation counts of main authors, institutions, journals, categories and countries are presented. Overall, the description shows the prominent role some authors as the principal authorities within the field, the predominance of United States in the citation counts as well as the high-impact journals in which the articles of this discipline are published. The most relevant implications of the findings are discussed in terms of future lines regarding the field of emotion regulation.

Keywords: Emotion regulation · Scientometric · Network analysis
Citation analysis

1 Introduction

Emotion regulation (ER) emerged in the last 15 years as one of the most studied constructs within the psychological realm. Although existing constructs aimed to address convergent domains (e.g. coping, mental control or emotional reactivity), the operationalization developed throughout the 90's constituted a turning point to examine how people seek to manage their emotional states. Indeed, ER is conceptualized as the processes deployed by a person or group of persons to explicitly or implicitly influence the experienced emotions to achieve desirable states or goals. Every person is at all times aiming at some extent to exert influence (implicit or explicit, automatic or

© ICST Institute for Computer Sciences, Social Informatics and Telecommunications Engineering 2018
P. Cipresso et al. (Eds.): MindCare 2018, LNICST 253, pp. 119–128, 2018.
https://doi.org/10.1007/978-3-030-01093-5_16

controlled) the experienced emotions, as well as when and how are elicited and expressed [1–3].

The proliferation of ER has been observed in a wide range of psychological branches, including experimental and applied research domains [4]. ER became a niche of interest due to diverse reasons, like the transversal and dimensional nature of the process, from clinical to non-clinical population [5] or being a cross-cultural construct [6]. Besides, it is of paramount importance to highlight the accurate but parsimonious operationalizations [7] that allow studying the construct at a research level with multiple psychophysiological, behavioral and subjective methods [8].

It is undoubtedly the case that ER has grown as a research field and some studies have yielded objective evidence on this issue. Illustrative examples are the increase of publications and citations [9], the presence of published papers in journals with the highest impact factor of each sub-discipline (e.g. in clinical psychology; [6, 9]) or the publication of several handbooks and books gathering the available evidence on the topic [4, 10, 11].

However, to better determine the real impact of ER on the psychological field, other indicators should be taken into account. In particular, bibliographic network analysis constitutes a paradigm that allows examining patterns and connections through the identification of authorities (authors, topics, journals, institutions, etc.) in a given scientific community [12]. Although there are different indicators that may show the scientific productivity of a research domain, unraveling which researchers are more cited in the field, with whom are they publishing (co-authorships) or in which journals are published these studies, may represent objective indicators to better weight and determine the current status of a specific field. Besides, it is a pristine platform to outline future challenges that the specific field of ER should face. Hence, the present study aims to present a computational bibliometric analysis to establish some of the defining features of the scientific proliferation of ER.

2 Methods

The input data for the analyses were retrieved from the scientific database Web of Science Core Collection, based on a topic search for Emotion Regulation ("emotion* regulation*") papers published during the whole timespan covered. The data were lastly updated on November 30, 2017. All the indexes that compose the Web of Science Core Collection were considered for the analysis. That is, Citation Indexes, Science Citation Index Expanded (SCI-EXPANDED) –1970-present, Social Sciences Citation Index (SSCI) –1970-present, Arts & Humanities Citation Index (A&HCI) – 1975-present, Conference Proceedings Citation Index- Science (CPCI-S) –1990- present, Conference Proceedings Citation Index- Social Science & Humanities (CPCI-SSH) –1990-present, Book Citation Index– Science (BKCI-S) –2009-present, Book Citation Index– Social Sciences & Humanities (BKCI-SSH) –2009-present, Emerging Sources Citation Index (ESCI) –2015-present, Chemical Indexes, Current Chemical Reactions (CCR-EXPANDED) –2009-present (Includes Institut National de la Propriete Industrielle structure data back to 1840), Index Chemicus (IC) –2009- present.

The resultant dataset contained a total of 11927. The bibliographic records consisted in diverse fields, such as author, title, abstract, and all the references (needed for the citation analysis). The research tool to visualize the networks was Cite space v.4.0. R5 SE (32 bit) 32 under Java Runtime v.8 update 91 (build 1.8.0_91-b15). One of the figures was done with Microsoft Excel.

3 Results

3.1 Number of Publications

First, an update of the number of publications in the field is presented. From the 90's on, when the term emotion regulation was popularized, an increasing number of articles are published yearly. While in the last years more than 1000 articles come out, previously to 2013 no year reached this threshold. In order to see that this growth is not a mere effect of the general increase of scientific publications [13], 3 other constructs that are convergent to emotion regulation, such as emotional intelligence, emotional reactivity and mental control were also included in the chart (Fig. 1).

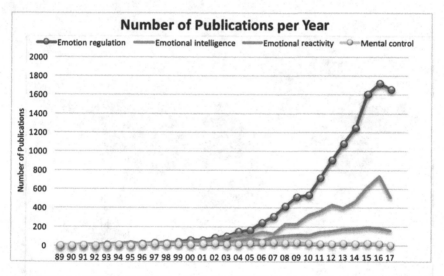

Fig. 1. Number of publications per year for Emotion regulation, emotional intelligence, emotional reactivity and mental control.

3.2 Country

In line with the predominance of the scientific production of the United States in many disciplines [14], the field of emotion regulation is not the exception to the rule. The total number of citations from the United States (5896) is more than the sum of the rest first 9 countries with most citation counts (4707).

122   J. Fernández-Álvarez et al.

Besides, as depicted in Table 1 and Fig. 2, almost all the citation counts belong to western countries. China is the only eastern country that appears among the first 10 and taking into consideration aggregated citations of the first 10 countries, it represents 4.01% of the total amount of citation counts.

Table 1. Citations for countries.

Heading level	Country
5896	United States
1082	Germany
703	Canada
595	England
548	Australia
511	The Netherlands
426	China
300	Spain
291	Italy
251	Switzerland

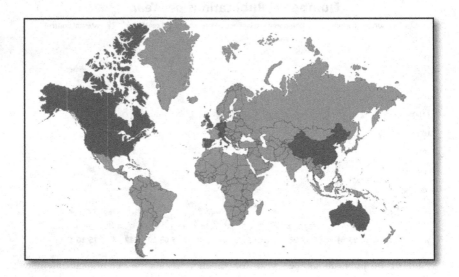

Fig. 2. Countries with more citations.

Figure 3 shows a highly centralized disposition as a whole since it is structured around a main focal point. United States constitutes undoubtedly the most important authority since it has clearly a central position, or in other words, shows higher degrees of connection. Additionally, it displays a bigger relative size in comparison to the rest of the countries. This centrality may also suggest that USA is cited by all countries, whereas other authorities, such as Germany, are mostly cited by a restricted community of countries.

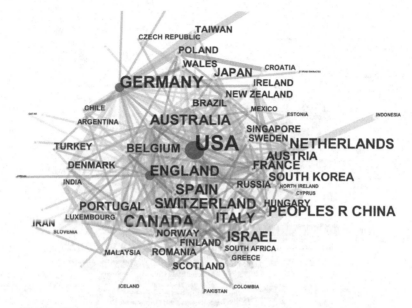

Fig. 3. Network of countries. It indicates the countries with more citations.

3.3 Institutions

In the same vein, United States shows a clear predominance regarding the most influential universities in terms of citation counts. Stanford University is the university with the highest number of citations, followed by University of Pittsburgh, Yale University and Harvard University, respectively. As Fig. 4 depicts, there are very few non-American universities placed in a central position (Table 2).

Table 2. Citation counts for institution.

Citation counts	Institution
284	Stanford University
208	University of Pittsburgh
190	Yale University
174	Harvard University
147	University of California Los Angeles
142	University of Illinois
141	Penn State University
141	University of Michigan
134	University of North Carolina
125	University of Toronto

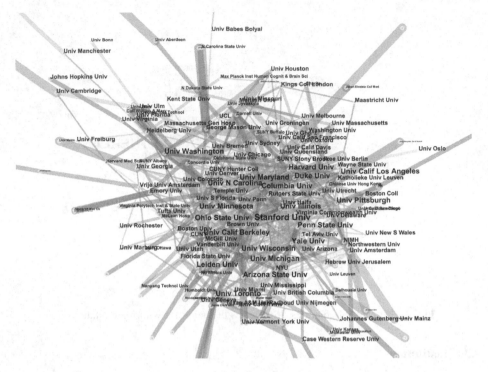

Fig. 4. Network of institutions.

3.4 Authors

The principal researcher in the topic in terms of citations is James Gross with 196 citation counts, followed by Kim Gratz and Matthew Tull with 65 and 62 citation counts, respectively. As long as 2003 constitutes the year of publication of the first and most used questionnaire of Emotion Regulation, the Emotion Regulation Questionnaire [15], a comparison of the authors up to 2003 and throughout all the years is presented. It is suggested that measuring the construct constitutes the cornerstone in order to study it at an applied level.

Whereas previous to 2003 almost all the authors are related to experimental psychology (Fig. 5), the network comprising all the years, depicts the central role played by more applied branches, particularly Clinical Psychology. Authors like Berking, Gratz, Tull, Hofmann or Joormann only appear in the last years. Moreover, the comparison of the two networks allows establishing the growing role of Gross as the main authority in the ER community (Fig. 6).

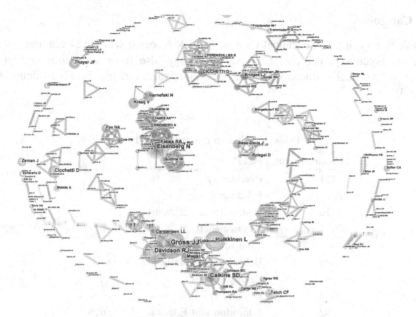

Fig. 5. Authors up to 2003.

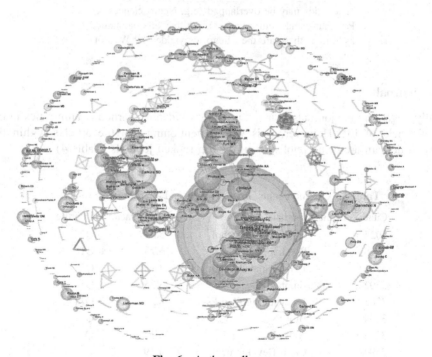

Fig. 6. Authors all years.

3.5   Categories

Psychology constitutes the truncal field within ER research with 7524 citation counts. However, psychiatry, neuroscience and neurology also have a predominant place. Interest in medical, educational and technological domains is also identifiable (Table 3).

Table 3. Citation counts for fields.

Citation counts	Field[a]
7524	Psychology
2691	Psychiatry
2426	Neurosciences & Neurology
2011	Neurosciences
591	Clinical Neurology
503	Behavioral sciences
361	Family studies
344	Physiology
292	Education and Educational research
271	Science & Technology

[a]The fields may be overlapped (e.g. Neurosciences & Psychiatry and Neurosciences), but they are maintained as long as these are the categories yielded by Web of Science.

3.6   Journals

Finally, regarding the journals, it is not possible to identify particular authorities in the specific field of ER. However, it is worth mentioning that the articles within the research domain are being published in the top ranked journals (Table 4).

Table 4. Citation counts, impact factor and quartile for journals.

Citation counts	Journals	Impact factor[b]	Quartile
6025	J. Pers Soc Psychol	5.017	Q1
4676	Psychol Bull	16.79	Q1
3581	J Abnormal Psychol	4.13	Q1
3502	Emotion	3.25	Q1
3363	J Consulting Clin Psychol	4.59	Q1
3294	Biol Psych	11.41	Q1
3214	Am J Psych	14.17	Q1
3194	Child Development	4.19	Q1
3144	Clin Psychol Rev	8.89	Q1
3065	Beh Res Ther	4.06	Q1

[b]Journal of Citation Report 2016

4 Discussion

Emotion Regulation shows to be a topic of great interest in the psychological realm. Although previous studies already described the exponential growth of publications in ER (e.g. [8]), two additional features can be identified within this new data. First, this exponential growth is maintained given that in the last 3 years the tendency of exponential growth continues. Furthermore, to our knowledge, this is the first data extracted from the Web Science Core Collection, which differently from Google Scholar does not include gray literature or other less exhaustively peer-reviewed evidence. Finally, another indicator of the proliferation of emotion regulation, not particularly in terms of quantity but of quality, is regarding the top ranked institutions and high impact factor journals in which the articles on the topic are published.

The fact that the total number of citations among the most productive countries are conducted in western countries, with a predominance of USA, Germany, England, Canada, The Netherlands and Australia is essential to grasp the bias that could be present in the scientific production within the ER field. Given the fact that emotion regulation has shown to be a highly culturally modulated construct, this is something important to be taken into account when generalizing the available results. Nevertheless, this predominance of USA and northern European countries is not specific of the field of emotion regulation, but of the scientific production in general [16].

In particular, United States has shown to be the most prominent authority, not only as a country but also due to the universities, authors and journals that are most cited. Undoubtedly, in terms of citation counts, James Gross is the main authority within the field. The publication of the first integrated review with an operationalized definition of the construct [1] constitutes a cornerstone of his contribution on the field. Besides, this author has contributed in a wide range of branches.

The fact that psychology is the central category within ER is rather logical as long as the construct of emotion is historically derived from philosophical studies but first scientifically addressed by the psychological science [17]. However, given that ER has shown to be particularly relevant as a transdiagnostic process in psychological and psychiatric disorders [5], branches like psychiatry, neurology and neuroscience account for an important percentage of the total citation counts.

Many aspects remain to be further studied within the field of ER and a more developed analysis of the current scientometrics may allow elucidating them. An illustrative example is to provide a conceptual distinction within the category *Emotion Regulation*. As long as it constitutes a construct that many researchers are willing to examine, both for real interest and for the attractiveness of studying burning issues, it is rather reasonable to ascertain that despite the initial consensus, the field is experiencing now a conceptual stretching. As a consequence, there is a lack of clarity regarding what does precisely constitute ER and what does not.

In this vein, through the identification of some key turning points (e.g. highly cited papers, new research categories or new research groups studying the construct), it may be possible to understand the evolution of the scientific production of ER as a field and thus to more specifically outline how to address the unexplored domains. Hence, apart from citation counts, other indicators (bursts, sigma or centrality) should be taken into account as well as more complex analysis should be carried out.

Acknowledgements. This work was supported by the Marie Skłodowska-Curie Innovative Training Network AffecTech (project ID: 722022) funded by the European Commission H2020.

References

1. Gross, J.: The emerging field of emotion regulation: an integrative review. Rev. Gen. Psychol. **2**(3), 271–299 (1998)
2. Zaki, J., Williams, W.C.: Interpersonal emotion regulation. Emotion **13**(5), 803–810 (2013)
3. Braunstein, L.B., Gross, J.J., Ochsner, K.N.: Explicit and implicit emotion regulation: a multi-level framework. Soc. Cogn. Affect. Neurosci. **12**(10), 1545–1557 (2017)
4. Gross, J.J.: Handbook of Emotion Regulation, 2nd edn. Guilford, New York (2014)
5. Aldao, A., Nolen-Hoeksema, N., Schweizer, S.: Emotion-regulation strategies across psychopathology: a meta-analytic review. Clin. Psychol. Rev. **30**(2), 217–237 (2010)
6. Ford, B.Q., Mauss, I.B.: Culture and emotion regulation. Curr. Opin. Psychol. **3**, 100–107 (2015)
7. Sheppes, G., Suri, G., Gross, J.: Emotion regulation and psychopathology. Annu. Rev. Clin. Psychol. **11**, 379–405 (2015)
8. Seeley, S.H., Garcia, E., Mennin, D.S.: Recent advances in laboratory assessment of emotion regulation. Curr. Opin. Psychol. **3**, 58–63 (2015)
9. Gross, J.J.: Emotion regulation: current status and future prospects. Psychol. Inq. **26**(1), 1–26 (2015)
10. Berking, M., Whitley, B.: Affect Regulation Training - A Practitioners' Manual. Springer, New York (2014). https://doi.org/10.1007/978-1-4939-1022-9
11. Kring, A.M., Sloan, D.: Emotion Regulation and Psychopathology A Transdiagnostic Approach to Etiology and Treatment. Guilford Press, New York (2010)
12. Scott, J., Carrington, P.J.: The Sage Handbook of Social Network Analysis. Sage, London (2011)
13. Larsen, P.O., von Ins, M.: The rate of growth in scientific publication and the decline in coverage provided by science citation index. Scientometrics **84**, 575–603 (2010)
14. Leydesdorff, L., Wagner, C.: Is the United States losing ground in science? A global perspective on the world science system. Scientometrics. **78**(1), 23–36. https://doi.org/10.1007/s11192-008-1830-4
15. Gross, J., John, O.P.: Individual differences in two emotion regulation processes: implications for affect, relationships, and well-being. J. Pers. Soc. Psychol. **85**(2), 348–362 (2003)
16. King, D.A.: The scientific impact of nations. Nature **430**(6997), 311–316 (2004)
17. Scarantino, A.: The philosophy of emotions and its impact on affective science. In: Barrett, L., Lewis, M., Haviland-Jones, J.M. (eds.) Handbook of Emotions, 4th edn, pp. 3–48. Guilford, New York (2016)

The *ActiveAgeing* Mobile App for Diabetes Self-management: First Adherence Data and Analysis of Patients' in-App Notes

Stefano Triberti[1(✉)], Sarah Bigi[2], Maria Grazia Rossi[3],
Amelia Caretto[4], Andrea Laurenzi[4], Nicoletta Dozio[4],
Marina Scavini[4], Enrico Pergolizzi[5], Alessandro Ozzello[5],
Silvia Serino[1,6], and Giuseppe Riva[1,6]

[1] Department of Psychology, Università Cattolica del Sacro Cuore, Milan, Italy
{stefano.triberti, silvia.serino,
giuseppe.riva}@unicatt.it
[2] Department of Linguistic Sciences and Foreign Literatures,
Università Cattolica del Sacro Cuore, Largo Gemelli 1, 20121 Milan, Italy
sarah.bigi@unicatt.it
[3] Institute of Philosophy of Language, FCSH Nova University of Lisbon,
Avenida de Berna 26, 1069-061 Lisbon, Portugal
mgrazia.rossi@fcsh.unl.pt
[4] Department of Endocrinology and Metabolic Diseases,
San Raffaele Scientific Institute, Università Vita-Salute, Via Olgettina 60,
20132 Milan, Italy
{caretto.amelia, laurenzi.andrea, dozio.nicoletta,
scavini.marina}@hsr.it
[5] Departmental Service of Endocrine Diseases and Diabetology, ASL TO3,
Stradale Fenestrelle 72, 10064 Pinerolo, Turin, Italy
{epergolizzi, aozzello}@aslto3.piemonte.it
[6] Applied Technology for NeuroPsychology Laboratory,
Istituto Auxologico Italiano, Via Magnasco 2, 20149 Milan, Italy

Abstract. The up-to-date treatment of diabetes often includes the adoption of technology (eHealth) to support patients' self-management. This contribution features first data on patients' usage of *ActiveAgeing*, a mobile app supporting daily self-management. Over 6 months, 15 elderly patients with type 2 diabetes (T2D) and 11 young women with gestational diabetes mellitus (GDM) received daily reminders to perform treatment activities, registered capillary glucose within the app, and added personal notes to explain abnormal values. While no differences emerged between the groups' glucose registrations, T2D patients were more likely to add notes. Sentiment analysis with the software Watson on T2D patients' notes and some selected notes are reported. Discussion highlights that notes may be used not only to explain abnormal data, but also to express emotions and confide personal information. eHealth presents opportunities not only for self-management, but also to empower and enrich trust between patients and health providers.

Keywords: eHealth · Self-care · Diabetes · Adherence · Personal notes
Patient engagement

© ICST Institute for Computer Sciences, Social Informatics and Telecommunications Engineering 2018
P. Cipresso et al. (Eds.): MindCare 2018, LNICST 253, pp. 129–138, 2018.
https://doi.org/10.1007/978-3-030-01093-5_17

1 Introduction

Global increase in the aging population, especially in Western countries, brings along a significant demand of care for chronic health conditions [1, 2], therefore requiring the elaboration, development and implementation of innovative ways to sustain care. Such instruments should not only be efficient and high-quality, but also cost-effective. This scenario sparked the rise of eHealth, or the use of new communication technologies to support healthcare [3, 4]. Indeed, technologies embedded in chronic patients' everyday life could assist them in disease management; for example, dedicated platforms can be used by patients to register and monitor treatment adherence (e.g., taking medications, adopting a more healthy lifestyle) [5–7], while computer mediated communication (CMC) and social media may be extraordinarily helpful in supporting communication between patients and different health care providers [8, 9], or even between patients themselves in order to encourage peer education and positive social influence. In addition to eHealth implementations to support treatment adherence and effectiveness, eHealth solutions have been proved useful also in the promotion of patient engagement [10, 11]. Specifically, new technologies are effective in terms of making patients more aware of their health status; equipping them with emotion-regulation resources to manage depression, stress and adverse emotional states; and, during advanced steps of the patient engagement process [12, 13], helping patients to recover their hobbies, passions and life goals despite the presence of a chronic disease.

In the field of eHealth implementations, diabetes, being one of the most common conditions has a huge interest. Indeed, diabetes has significant impact on patient's everyday life. First, this disease requires numerous factors to be constantly monitored (e.g., glycemic values, weight, adherence to medications); secondly, it also notably affects quality of life because the disease management necessitates for specific, daily activities to be timely performed (e.g., insulin administration, diet changes, frequent medical consultations).

In this context, numerous technologies have been developed in order to empower patients' daily disease management, however, only few have been tested. The present contribution includes an analysis of the first implementation of *ActiveAgeing*, a mobile app for diabetes self-management.

1.1 The *ActiveAgeing* Application

Among currently available mobile applications for the control of diabetes, few seem to include specific educational functions. It is often not clear what kind of interactional and clinical model they are based on, nor if they have been tested for beneficial effects on users' self-management skills and self-efficacy levels [14, 15].

The design of the *ActiveAgeing* application (henceforth, AA app) takes into account the tenets of the Chronic Care Model [16], the conditions for patient engagement [11, 12] and the clinical goals for patients with diabetes [17]. Among these goals, self-management skills are very important, as they guarantee that patients – through their healthy behaviors – will be able to maintain optimal control and avoid long-term complications as well as manage acute situations of mild hyperglycaemia or hypoglycaemia. Indeed, acute episodes can seriously affect patients' quality of life and represent a significant burden for healthcare systems. Self-management skills are supported by a correct understanding of the problem, the awareness of the solutions available and the possibility to put them into practice; in other words, by critical thinking skills. However, patients with diabetes have infrequent and short outpatient clinic appointments and only during the consultations do they have the opportunity to critically think about their condition, correlate behaviors with parameters and discuss possible solutions for very specific management problems, and receive feedback by their doctors.

Thus, the AA app was developed as a tool to be integrated within the therapeutic alliance between doctors and patients and aiming at increasing patients' awareness of their condition and their decision-making autonomy. To reach these goals, the app needs to be used by doctor and patient in a complementary way.

The app receives input data from two sources: (1) the doctor, who performs the setup together with the patient when the app is installed on the patient's smartphone. In this phase, individualized parameter ranges are set and lifestyle information is provided; (2) the patient, who records clinical parameters according to the schedule recommended by the doctor. The data are saved on a web platform that is accessible to both doctor and patient through the patient's phone number and a password, set by the patient. The app then functions by comparing the data recorded by patients with the data entered during the setup phase and by providing immediate feedback in the form of textual messages, graphs and symbols. The messages provide reward, encouragement, they bring the patient's attention to parameters that are not within the set ranges, provide suggestions for coping with a potentially risky situation and suggestions for finding the causes of such situations. It is in particular in this last case that the app points out the possibility to take notes about what could have caused a certain parameter to be out of range. Notes can be inserted by typing in a dedicated space whatever patients feel is relevant. Apart from realizing an important tracking function that is very useful when the values are then discussed during the visit in the outpatient clinic with the doctor, the act itself of writing comments about such values can have an impact on the capacity of patients to actively reflect and think about their own health condition.

1.2 Objectives

The AA app has been used by two groups of individuals, namely elderly with established type 2 diabetes (T2D) and young pregnant women with a new diagnosis of gestational diabetes mellitus (GDM). These groups, intrinsically different for age and sex, were compared for adherence measures.

To address the research question, "how do patients use the notes function within the app, or, what information and meanings do they convey through it?" we analyzed the available patients' notes.

2   Method

2.1   Sample

Results discussed in the next section refer to patients recruited between 01/01/2017 and 31/08/2017. In total, 26 patients accepted to participate and were enrolled in this study: 15 T2D patients with a median age of 69 (range 65–73) and 11 GDM patients with a median age of 37 (range 34–40). They were recruited in two different hospitals in northern Italy. Specifically, GDM patients were recruited at San Raffaele Hospital (Milan, Italy), while T2D patients were recruited both at San Raffaele Hospital (Milan, Italy) and at ASL TO3 - Pinerolo (Turin, Italy). The study was approved by the Ethics Committees of both participating institutions (Protocol No. 105/2016 DRI006 and 0005047, respectively).

Inclusion criteria for both groups of participants were: diagnosis of diabetes, clinical parameters that showed difficulties of self-management, non-satisfactory clinical profiles, therapeutic prescriptions (tablets or insulin), and ability to use a smartphone. All participants spoke and read Italian fluently.

2.2   Procedures

Patients meeting the inclusion criteria were recruited by endocrinologists during a regularly scheduled consultation, after receiving all relevant information about the study. In this phase, clinical parameters were collected by the endocrinologists, who also proposed and discussed the app setup with patients. In a second phase, patients signed a written informed consent and met with the researchers from Università Cattolica del Sacro Cuore of Milan (Italy) to install the app and be instructed about its functioning. Apps were set up according to the endocrinologist's recommendations discussed with patients during the consultation.

2.3   Data Preparation and Analysis

The present paper reports three kinds of data: statistical analyses on adherence; sentiment analysis on patients' in-app notes; and, selected patients' in-app notes with a significant anecdotal value.

First, adherence data have been computed to compare T2D and GDM patients. Each patient had a specific treatment plan to follow depending on his/her diabetes diagnosis. Each patient had also a specific self-monitoring of blood glucose (SMBG) regimen to follow according to endocrinologists' prescriptions. By comparing the total number of SMBGs each patient should have performed and the actual number they recorded in the app, the researchers were able to compute for each patient a percentage value of actual measurements against ideal measurements. This value has been labeled 'Adherence' as a measure of patient's commitment to self-monitoring via the mobile app.

The second analysis focused on in-app notes; these were intended as a resource for patients to add more information regarding abnormal capillary glucose (e.g., too high or too low glycemic values), illness state or lifestyle. Considering the total number of notes present in the database, a new variable has been computed for each patient: 0 = patient added zero notes; 1 = patient added 1 to 5 notes; 2 = patient added 5 to 10 notes; 3 = patient added 10 to 15 notes; 4 = patient added more than 15 notes. This variable is intended to give information about the patient overlooking, just trying, occasionally or frequently using, or being seriously committed to the notes function.

Moreover, as some T2D patients included a high number of notes within the app, it was interesting to analyze what kind of information was present in them. However, in-app notes were not adequate to perform rigorous textual analysis; as previously said, some patients added no notes or a very low number of them, while others made an extremely assiduous use of this function; moreover, notes are extremely variable in their content, in that sometimes they are composed by just a couple of words, while other times they include elaborate sentences, vivid descriptions and narrations. Therefore, the researchers decided to employ a sentiment analysis. Sentiment analysis software are able to analyze texts in order to extract emotional lexicon and its frame of reference, as well as to attribute a global positive/negative value to the text and quantify existent discrete emotions [18]. For the present study, the researchers employed the IBM software Watson (https://www.ibm.com/watson/), which includes advanced features for Natural Language Processing/Understanding and Sentiment Analysis [19, 20]. In order to use the software, the researchers have translated patients' notes in English maintaining the highest possible adherence to literary meaning; then, T2D patients' notes with more than one sentence available in notes were included in the analysis (GDM patients' notes were generally too rare and brief and the researchers decided they were not adequate for sentiment analysis).

Finally, some selected in-app notes by patients will be reported and their anecdotal value, useful to understand patients' experience, will be briefly discussed.

3   Results

The three types of results will be reported in three subsections.

3.1   Adherence Data

A t-test has been performed comparing T2D patients and GDM patients on the Adherence variable. Although T2D patients (M = 81, DS = 75.5) were generally more adherent than GDM patients (M = 58.18, DS = 31.5) in registering glycemic data, the analysis reached no significance: $t(1,25) = .933$, $p = .363$. It has to be noted that the number of SMBGs required for individuals with type 2 diabetes was on average 4 per week and the observation period spanned several months, whereas the SBGMs required for individuals with GD were at least 4 per day and the observation period was limited to 3 months.

For what regard the number of in-app notes, as this variable is based on an ordinal scale, a non-parametric statistic (Mann-Whitney test) was used to compare T2D and GDM patients. T2D patients were significantly more likely than GDM patients (M = 1.66, SD = 1.6 vs M = 0.36, SD = 0.5, respectively) to leave personal notes within the app ($Z = -2.160$, $U = 43.500$, $p = .041$, $r = .42$).

3.2   Sentiment Analysis

Indeed, the researchers noticed that, although the majority of the notes included information about food and life activities (because notes were especially intended to explain abnormal glycemic values), there were occasional references to emotional states and personal confidences (see next section for notable examples of patients' notes). Table 1 features individual patients' total number of words in the notes and the corresponding sentiment and emotional values attributed to them by Watson's analysis.

Table 1. Patients' total number of words in notes and corresponding values attributed by Watson's sentiment/emotional analysis. On numbering: patients were originally listed in the database based on the presence of notes, for this reason their numbering is consequential. Patient 7 has been excluded because he added just one note of a couple of words.

Patient	Total words	Sentiment (Positive/Negative)	Joy	Anger	Disgust	Sadness	Fear
1	27	0.88	0.80	0.01	0.01	0.07	0.04
2	133	0.29	0.48	0.08	0.53	0.15	0.06
3	70	−0.75	0.52	0.08	0.09	0.18	0.07
4	30	−0.16	0.61	0.11	0.10	0.13	0.06
5	170	−0.28	0.47	0.11	0.47	0.15	0.48
6	73	0.60	0.66	0.05	0.09	0.08	0.06
8	156	−0.77	0.24	0.15	0.52	0.58	0.19
9	69	0.29	0.48	0.08	0.53	0.15	0.06

It is important to take into account that these data should be interpreted with caution. Their inclusion in this study is not meant to constitute a rigorous analysis of patients' emotions, on the contrary they are intended as clues about the actual presence of emotional contents in patients' notes. Indeed, all patients obtain notable scores in joy in that the majority of notes are written with a positive and proactive attitude; also, explicitly happy and humorous comments are present. Occasional scores in sadness and fear are probably related to explicit statements about illness and the disease, while disgust scores may be related to the numerous food words associated with shame/regret for having eaten too much and therefore having negatively influenced glycemic values.

3.3   Patients' Selected Notes

Reporting some patients' notes is interesting to understand how this function of the app has been actually used and intended by the patients. Table 2 includes some selected notes from the app database, along with reference to patients (Italian original text and English translation).

Note (a) represents the majority of notes present in the database; this is how most of the patients' notes look like. As users were invited to include notes when glycemic values were above the limit suggested by the clinician, most of the notes feature possible justification for high values, therefore they describe food intakes prior to measurement.

Table 2. Selected patients' in-app notes.

Reference in text	Patient, note number	Content (Italian, English)
(a)	Patient 2, note 11	"A mezzogiorno ho mangiato insalata, due uova, un panino e una fetta di crostata e un bicchiere di vino" "At noon I ate salad, two eggs, one sandwich and a slice of pie and a glass of wine"
(b)	Patient 1, note 1	"È la prima volta che la misurazione si mantiene quasi su valori std. Infatti 136 al mattino non rispecchia i miei valori precedenti. Sono contento!" "It is the first time that the measurement is almost on standard values. Indeed 136 in the morning does not mirror my previous values. I'm happy!"
(c)	Patient 9, note 5	"Ho mangiato in mattinata perché mi sentivo vuoto" "I ate during the morning because I felt empty"
(d)	Patient 4, notes 1, 2, 5, 7	"Pranzi in Valle d'Aosta un po' pesanti" "Inizio ferie al mare" "Fine ferie" "Colpa delle ferie" "Lunches in Aosta Valley a little heavy" "Starting holidays at the sea" "Ending holidays" "It's holidays' fault"
(e)	Patient 9, note 7	"Vado in ferie torno il 30/05" "Going on holidays will be back on May, 30"

Differently, the other notes selected for the table show how patients sometimes used the app function to describe more intimate, confidential and/or emotional information. For example, note (b) accompanied a positive measurement, therefore it was an autonomous initiative by the patient (it was not suggested by the app). It includes a specific positive statement in that the patient wants to share his satisfaction for having reached a personal goal. Differently, note (c) features an ambiguous statement that may have an important emotional value. Indeed, both in Italian and English "feeling empty" may simply refer to feeling hunger, but it is an interesting choice of words that could also refer to sadness. Indeed, here the patient decided to not simply describe what he ate, nor to explicitly say that he was hungry, but he felt it was important to report a psychological sensation that moved him to eat outside of normal meal times.

The notes reported in (d) are quite interesting; the patient is basically using the notes app function as a small personal diary. He records the duration of his holidays with personal judgments instead of mere food or activities description, almost as if it was important for him to establish a personal dialogue with the clinician about what is happening in his life. Indeed, these notes constitute a small narration including context, events and emotional reactions.

In this sense note (e), wrote by the same author of note (c), is similar because it does not include justification of a problematic glycemic value: it is the last note of patient 9. Here, the patient is using the notes app function to say that his holidays are about to start. As the patient apparently foresees to be busy with holiday activities (or possibly prone to eat more than usual in the holiday context), he thinks that it is important to notify to the clinician about his life activities and maybe to justify why he will not write notes anymore during a busy period.

4 Discussion

This research compared patients with type 2 diabetes and gestational diabetes mellitus in their use of *ActiveAgeing*, a mobile application supporting self-care for diabetes. Statistical analyses show that there were no significant differences among T2D and GDM patients in the use of the app to register glycemic values, on the contrary both groups were generally satisfactorily adherent to the use of the app, thus empowering their self-care. Differently, T2D patients were significantly more likely to use the app's notes function, namely the opportunity to add personal written notes to glycemic/weight registration in order to explain anomalies. According to this result, T2D patients may be more engaged in the technology use in that they show personal initiative and the intention to help the clinician understand their health state. This could be related to type 2 diabetes' specific characteristics, i.e. a lifelong condition with high demands for daily self-engagement in care, with infrequent contacts with health professionals in a phase of life where other commitments might be reduced; on the other hand, women with GDM are pregnant and engaged in self and unborn child care, with frequent contacts with health professionals and an active daily life.

Secondarily, in-app notes by eight T2D patients have been analyzed. Watson's analysis showed that emotional aspects can be found in the notes, so their content cannot be reduced to "cold" reports of food intakes or care-related activities. Some interesting notes by the patients have been reported in order to highlight meaningful examples. It should be specified that such data cannot be generalized to a population, instead they should be considered as anecdotal information useful to understand the potentials of the *ActiveAgeing* app. Indeed, some patients showed a meaningful personal initiative by using the app function beyond its actual scope, which was adding details to possible abnormal glucose values (e.g., too high glycemic values). Sometimes, the notes function has been used to express emotions ("I'm happy!"), to write a "small personal diary", or to notify about life activities that may interfere with the app usage, as if it were a direct contact/appointment with the health provider ("I'm going on holidays, I will be back on May, 30"). Such examples show that the app's notes function could be developed further in order to constitute an actual tool for empowering the patient/doctor relationship, because patients actually use this affordance to express emotion and convey complex communicative intentions. Such a behavior actually transcends the concept of treatment adherence and hints at the one of patient engagement, or the proactive involvement of the patient in his/her own care plan [21, 22].

5 Conclusion

The present study showed that the *ActiveAgeing* app was generally successful in helping diabetes patients to monitor their own health. Preliminary data show that patients with type 2 diabetes were more likely to use the notes function to add details on their state, and also that they sometimes used such function to express emotions and convey complex communicative intentions. The main limitations of this study are related to the small number of subjects, and the different characteristics of the groups with regard to age and sex, which may act as confounding variables. Moreover, it should be taken into account that the interpretations of T2D patients' in-app notes are purely anecdotal and should not be generalized to a population of patients, nor used to conclude strong inferences. Future studies on eHealth instruments should deepen the opportunities for empowering the communication between patient and clinician, in order to make use of self-care apps beyond their mere treatment adherence and health monitoring functions. Nevertheless, these should be tailored to specific patient group characteristics.

Acknowledgments. The study reported in this publication was supported by a grant from Università Cattolica del Sacro Cuore of Milan. The title of the grant is: "Progetto di ricerca d'interesse per l'Ateneo, Linea D.3.2, Anno 2014" for the project titled "Tecnologia Positiva e Healthy Ageing", PI: Giuseppe Riva; and also, by Fondazione Cariplo within the project "Active Aging and Healthy Living."

References

1. Busse, R., Blümel, M., Scheller-Kreinsen, D., Zentner, A.: Tackling Chronic Disease in Europe: Strategies, Interventions and Challenges. Observatory Studies Series No 20. World Health Organization, Copenhagen (2010)
2. Triberti, S., Barello, S.: The quest for engaging AmI: patient engagement and experience design tools to promote effective assisted living. J. Biomed. Inform. **63**, 150–156 (2016)
3. Eysenbach, G.: Medicine 2.0: social networking, collaboration, participation, apomediation, and openness. J. Med. Internet Res. **10**, 3 (2008)
4. Gaddi, A., Capello, F.: The debate over eHealth. In: Gaddi, A., Capello, F., Manca, M. (eds.) eHealth Care and Quality of Life. Springer, Heidelberg (2014). https://doi.org/10.1007/978-88-470-5253-6_1
5. Boulos, M.N.K., Wheeler, S., Tavares, C., Jones, R.: How smartphones are changing the face of mobile and participatory healthcare: an overview, with example from eCAALYX. Biomed. Eng. Online **10**, 24 (2011)
6. Eland-de Kok, P., van Os-Medendorp, H., Vergouwe-Meijer, A., Bruijnzeel-Koomen, C., Ros, W.: A systematic review of the effects of e-health on chronically ill patients. J. Clin. Nurs. **20**, 2997–3010 (2011)
7. Mohr, D.C., Burns, M.N., Schueller, S.M., Clarke, G., Klinkman, M.: Behavioral intervention technologies: evidence review and recommendations for future research in mental health. Gen. Hosp. Psychiat. **35**(4), 332–338 (2013)
8. Dedding, C., van Doorn, R., Winkler, L., Reis, R.: How will e-health affect patient participation in the clinic? A review of e-health studies and the current evidence for changes in the relationship between medical professionals and patients. Soc. Sci. Med. **72**, 49–53 (2011)
9. Glick, T.H., Moore, G.T.: Time to learn: the outlook for renewal of patient-centred education in the digital age. Med. Educ. **35**(5), 505–509 (2001)
10. Barello, S., Triberti, S., Graffigna, G., Libreri, C., Serino, S., Hibbard, J., Riva, G.: eHealth for patient engagement: a systematic review. Front. Psychol. **6**, 2013 (2016). https://doi.org/10.3389/fpsyg.2015.02013
11. Graffigna, G., Barello, S., Triberti, S.: Patient Engagement: A Consumer-Centered Model to Innovate Healthcare. De Gruyter Open, Berlin (2015)

12. Graffigna, G., Barello, S., Bonanomi, A., Lozza, E.: Measuring patient engagement: development and psychometric properties of the patient health engagement (PHE) scale. Front. Psychol. **6**, 274 (2015)
13. Graffigna, G., Barello, S., Libreri, C., Bosio, C.A.: How to engage type-2 diabetic patients in their own health management: implications for clinical practice. BMC Public Health **14**, 648 (2014)
14. Rossi, M.G., Bigi, S.: mHealth for diabetes support: a systematic review of apps available on the Italian market. mHealth **4**, 3–16 (2017)
15. Rossi, M.G., Bigi, S.: Weak educational components in mHealth devices for diabetes support available on the Italian market. J. Diabetes Sci. Technol. **10**(5), 1199 (2016)
16. Coleman, K., Austin, B.T., Brach, C., Wagner, E.H.: Evidence on the chronic care model in the new millennium. Health Affair **28**(1), 75–85 (2009)
17. Alberti, K.G.M.M., Zimmet, P., Shaw, J.: International diabetes federation: a consensus on Type 2 diabetes prevention. Diabetic Med. **24**(5), 451–463 (2007)
18. Yi, J., Nasukawa, T., Bunescu, R., Niblack, W.: Sentiment analyser: extraction sentiments about a given topic using natural language processing techniques. In: IEEE International Conference on Data Mining (ICDM), pp. 427–434 (2003)
19. Ferrucci, D.A.: Introduction to "This is Watson". IBM J. Res. Develop. **56**(3.4), 1:1–1:15 (2012)
20. High, R.: The era of cognitive systems: an inside look at IBM Watson and how it works. Int. Bus. Mach. Corporation **1**(1), 1–14 (2012)
21. Barello, S., Graffigna, G., Vegni, E.: Patient engagement as an emerging challenge for healthcare services: mapping the literature. Nurs. Res. Pract. **2012**, 1–7 (2012)
22. Graffigna, G., Barello, S., Triberti, S., Wiederhold, B.K., Bosio, A.C., Riva, G.: Enabling eHealth as a pathway for patient engagement: a toolkit for medical practice. Stud. Health Technol. Inform. **199**, 13–21 (2014)

Tools and Technologies for Patients and Caregivers Engagement: A Qualitative Analysis of Health Professionals' Attitudes and Day-to-Day Practice

Serena Barello[(✉)] and Guendalina Graffigna

Department of Psychology, Università Cattolica del Sacro Cuore di Milano,
L. go Gemelli 1, 20123 Milan, Italy
serena.barello@unicatt.it

Abstract. As patient engagement cannot be achieved without health professionals co-operation and agreement, attention to the clinicians' views and attitudes about patient engagement is essential in order to deepen potential enablers and barriers for its implementation. This qualitative study aimed to identify health professionals' attitudes towards patient engagement and the perceived hindrances and facilitators to the implementation of the patient engagement strategies in their routine practice with a particular focus of health information technologies for patient engagement. It identifies the dimensions underlying patient engagement realization, namely clinicians' *"Meanings and attitudes towards patient engagement"*, *"practical experience of patient engagement"*, and *"being a health professional in the era of patient engagement"*, as well as highlights the fashion in which these dimensions operate will either activate or inhibit patient engagement innovation. Finally, the study highlighted the great potential of health technologies to support patient engagement if they are enablers of the patient-clinician relationship and not replace it.

Keywords: Patient engagement · Health professionals · Professional identity Technologies

1 Introduction

Healthcare systems in Europe are currently confronted with the rising incidence of chronic illness. This epidemiological shift is challenging the traditional healthcare delivery models largely to provide acute care and manage infectious diseases [1, 2]. The paternalistic approach to healthcare, where health professionals make all of the decisions with little or no input from the patient, has evolved over the past 20 years towards a patient-centered care model that aims to personalize care according to individual patients' needs, values, and experiences [3–7].

As patient engagement cannot be achieved without health professionals co-operation and agreement, attention to the clinicians' attitudes about patient engagement is essential in order to deepen potential enablers and barriers for its implementation. Moreover, although patients gain skills from within and outside the healthcare system,

© ICST Institute for Computer Sciences, Social Informatics and Telecommunications Engineering 2018
P. Cipresso et al. (Eds.): MindCare 2018, LNICST 253, pp. 139–149, 2018.
https://doi.org/10.1007/978-3-030-01093-5_18

their interaction with the health practitioners who have them in charge remains one of the main resource for encouraging their active engagement in the medical course [5, 6]. Without collecting the clinicians' perspective on this concept, interventions to optimize chronic patient engagement are at risk of being misdirected and achieving suboptimal clinical and quality improvement outcomes. Moreover, the last decades have assisted to an actual technological revolution that deeply restructured the ways people search and use information for healthcare purposes. For these reasons, new technologies are fundamental resources to fostering patient engagement in chronic care settings. At the same time, these tools need to be accepted and effectively used by both patients and their care providers [8, 9]. According to these premises, we performed an exploratory qualitative study, aimed to identify health professionals' belief and attitudes towards the concept of patient engagement and the perceived hindrances and facilitators to the implementation of the patient engagement strategies in their routine practice with a particular focus of health information technologies for patient engagement.

2 Methods

2.1 Study Design and Setting

We conducted an exploratory qualitative study between November 2015 and February 2016 analyzing data from focus groups and semi-structured individual interviews involving HCPs from a multi-disciplinary perspective. Participants provided written informed consent to participate in the study. The Ethics committee approved this consent procedure.

2.2 Population

In order to obtain a cross-section of health professionals operating in the chronic field, we sought a heterogeneous and multidisciplinary sample, stratified by clinical area (diabetes, cardiovascular disease, pulmonary disease, oncology, neurology), discipline (doctors, nurses, psychologists, physiotherapists), setting of clinical practice (hospital and private practice), age (<45 years versus >45 years), and gender. Finally, we purposively accessed health professionals of different level of experience.

2.3 Data Collection and Analysis

Focus groups took place interviews were conducted between March and June 2017. Before the conduction of focus groups and interviews, participants received an information sheet and signed an informed consent for being included in the study. Two researchers (SB and GG) conducted focus groups and interviews. Focus groups and interviews were audio-recorded and transcribed verbatim.

3 Results

3.1 Characteristics and Descriptions of Focus Groups and Interviews

Overall, N = 66 HCPs participated in the study. *Four* focus groups were conducted with a total of 38 participants: (a) physicians (N = 11); (b) nurses (N = 6); other healthcare professionals (N = 22, including 14 psychologist, 4 sociologists, 1 health educators, 1 physiotherapists). The mean duration of the focus groups was 117 min and the mean amount of female participants of the focus was 65%. Additionally, 28 interviews with a total of 24 physicians and 4 nurses were carried out. The mean duration of the interviews was 52 min. 39% participants were female.

3.2 Qualitative Analysis

Three main themes were identified: *health professionals meanings and attitudes* towards chronic patient engagement, *practical experiences* with patient engagement and *being a health professional in the era of patient engagement*.

3.2.1 Meanings and Attitudes Towards Patient Engagement

HCPs' Perspective on Patient Engagement. There was almost unanimous agreement among the involved HCPs that patients should play an active role in their own healthcare. Generally, health professionals embraced the value and highlighted the ethical urgency of patient engagement policies because they felt patients themselves are more and more demanding for higher levels of engagement in their care. Participants underlined that, although doctors can manage the medical aspect of a chronic condition, patients need to have an active role in making lifestyle changes in order to reduce possible complications and to chose their preferred care pathway. Views on the extent to which patients should take responsibility over their healthcare process varied and suggested different underlying perspectives on the meaning attached to this concept. Notably, patient engagement in the health professionals' representations ranged from a more passivizing logic to a more empowering one. Particularly, HCPs referred to engaged patients as ones *"adhering to what they have been told to do"*, to *"openly communicating doubts and fears to clinicians"*, to *"discussing with the healthcare team about care expectations and treatment decisions"*, to *"prompting HCPs about their care practices and identifying shared wellness goals"*. This active engagement was termed as patients being a *"...partner in their healthcare"*. Particularly, some HCPs described the concept of patient engagement as *"improving the patients' knowledge and self-efficacy and educating them so that they can take steps themselves"*. This conceptualization mainly refer to the educative component of the therapeutic relationship which should aims to give patient the necessary skills and competences to become expert in their health and disease management. *"Patient engagement...what I understand about that is that there is the need to inform patients about their health condition and what we can do to manage it. Secondly we have to discuss these information with patients and check their understanding and if the therapeutic options might fits them". (Cardiologist, ambulatory practice).*

Many participants associated patient engagement with *"patients asking questions and acquiring knowledge"* about their care process. This conceptualization mainly refers to the patients' communicative behaviors during the medical encounter and to their level of proactivity in sharing concerns and actively search for information by the doctor. *"I think that people can be more involved if they get the opportunity to say something themselves, to ask questions they feel relevant. Not only about their medical problems but also about their quality of life. For this reason a HCP should make time to listen to them". (Neurologist, hospital).*

Although HCPs valued a paradigmatic shift towards an increased patient engagement in the care process, their comments suggested that this was not necessarily straightforward and it can take confidence to be able to share some of the control and responsibility with the patient. *"I think that there is a danger of putting too much responsibility on the patient to make clinical decisions about their condition without the adequate support...But, on the other hand, there a many patients that want to be told what to do and how. In some ways it is really difficult because we need to assess the individuals, you can't just do a change of rules and policies". (Cardiologist, hospital).*

Positive and Negative Outcomes of Patient Engagement
Participants generally agree on patients' adherence to medication as the most important expected positive outcome of patient engagement, along with significant improvements of doctor-patient relationship. Engaging patients allows improvements in *"honest and trust communication with patients"* who become, in their turn, increasingly confortable to question HCPs about their care and disease control. *"An engaged patient generally feels better and can do his/her life in a normal way...that's because he can adhere to medical prescriptions and – as a consequence – his/her quality of life improves". (pneumologist).* Engaged patients, in the HCPs perspectives, are more aware of their health conditions and are more able to search for relevant information and appropriately ask for medical support when needed. *"Engaging patients are a great resource for us (doctor) because they are more informed and they understand their health conditions and why I have to suggest them to do something or to avoid something else...they understand why certain drugs have to be taken or why they should follow a healthy diet...for these reason they can effectively self-manage "without" us..." (diabetologist).*

Many of the participants also reported patient engagement as a proxy of patient satisfaction with the received care; moreover, it would reduce patients' worries and litigation and increase patient's understanding of disease and treatment choices. Finally, one HCP refer that: *"I definitely think that engage patients is the best solution because when we should communicate that something is not going well they understand and they are much more open to redefine the therapeutic goals..." (oncologist).*

On the other hand, HCPs referred that their own job satisfaction would improve as well by engaging patients in the care process. They consider patient engagement as a continuing challenge and thought it would give them more background information about patients, which would enable them to collect patients' needs and preferences better. *"Engaging patients is just a satisfaction for us (doctors) because it allows to set the ground for an more satisfying relationship with them" (neurologist).*

Finally, patient engagement was perceived as a mean to make more equitable the consultation in terms of duties and responsibilities. *"People tend to get better control with their disease, probably a better regulation when they are engaged. And if they know what is going on and are in control over they health status, well...when the patient we have in front is really engaged we are in two to remember what is going to happen"* (diabetologist).

Concerning the potential negative outcomes of engaging patients, some HCPs referred anxiety about patient engagement, for example because consultation might become longer or people would ask too much questions. *"I think that engaging patients might have some dark sides...when patients are involved might require much more time because they are more aware and tend to ask a lot of questions...but we have really little time...just five minutes for each of them"* (cardiologist). Despite patient engagement being advocated by participants concerns was also expressed that this practice might results in patients becoming too much confident and avoid seeking help when necessary. Responses suggested that HCPs themselves needed to feel in control in order to fulfill their professional role and responsibilities.

3.2.2 Practical Experiences with Patient Engagement

Facilitators and barriers towards patient engagement. Barriers to the implementation of patient engagement were mentioned at different levels. Key barriers were grouped under three analytical categories: (a) *How the healthcare organization functions?* (b) *What happens during the patient-clinician relationship?* (c) *Who is the patient?*

(a) *How does the healthcare organization function?*

With regard to *organizational aspect of clinical practice*, HCPs reported that in their perceptions they have *too limited time* to effectively engage patients. This lack of time for consultation would limit the possibility of clinicians to adequately inform patients and also to give them the right space and time to ask questions, raise concerns and discuss issues with their clinicians. Conversely, adequate time for discussion can facilitate patient engagement in making shared treatment plans and can afford opportunities for high quality relationship building and more patient-centered communication. *"We have problems of timing...if you have 15 min for each visit and in this 15 min you have to discuss the clinical exams, set the therapeutic plan, write down the drugs prescriptions...12 min have just gone away...and only 3 min are available to speak with the patient..."* (diabetologist).

Another important theme belonging to the organizational aspects is the *continuity of care*: HCPs refers that poor continuity of care is a major barriers to patient engagement as chronic care requires strong coordination among health services and providers who have in charge the patients' management. Many clinicians, in this regards, expressed concerns that care is becoming more and more fragmented, thus threatening their own ability to make sense of the patients' needs and develop a partnership relationship. HPSs, in this regard, advocate the need for a case manager that helps the care team to guarantee to the patient the needed care coordination. *"How can patients take the most benefit from their healthcare if they don't perceive a fil rouge along their care process? If they feel that each HP is an interlocutor completely detached from the others?"* (cardiologist).

(b) *What happens during the patient-clinician relationship?*

Generally, participants agreed that the way in which health care professionals interact and communicate with patients could affect patient engagement in health care. Health care professionals who respond positively to patients' needs and views and who provide feedbacks to patients concerns can increase patient engagement. Conversely, health care professionals who are dismissive towards the patients' concerns can decrease the level of patient engagement. *"It (patient engagement) strongly depends on the doctor...if he/she is not available to listen to the patient...engagement can't occur..." (oncologist); "You should be open and available to give the patient the space...communication is fundamental" (cardiologist).*

A major barrier relates to the traditional presumptions and expectations about the patient role in the care process where normal patients are passive and expect clinicians to make decisions. HCPs often report that explicit encouragement to be involved in the clinical process could be a facilitator for patient to take an active role in their care; some patients, indeed, might feel they do not have the right to be involved in their healthcare. *"Some people need to be stimulated more. By nature they can be inclined not to ask to much to their doctors, to agree always what the doctor says. They are not used to be interactive with us..." (doctor, oncologist, hospital).*

Another factor frequently discussed by HCPs was the presence or absence of trust within the clinical relationship. A trusting relationship is considered by the majority of clinicians as one of the most powerful precursor of patient engagement: trust makes patients more willing to ask questions, report their concerns or troubles with the disease management. *"When you succeed to build a relationship based on mutual trust you have won the match with that patient. Without trust nothing will happen...you risk to lose the patient...." (doctor, cardiologist, ambulatory).* Also the use of the medical lexicon could be a barrier to patient engagement. Patients feel that clinicians are taking "another language" and may misinterpret the content of the communication. Conversely, "layman terms" might facilitate the patient understanding and also allows them to intervene in the conversation. *"Clinician should speak the language of their patients. The use of medical terms protect ourselves from the patients' questions and fears...but it is not useful in the long term" (doctors oncologist, hospital).* Most factors related to interpersonal characteristics of the patient-doctor relation could be modifiable by supporting positive attitudes towards patient engagement among both patients and clinicians. In this sense, both medical and patient education on this topic is reported by the clinician involved in the study as a fundamental strategy to promote a cultural shift towards the value of engaging patients in their medical course and emphasizing their role and responsibilities over their health management. *"I think that not only technical education is needed by clinicians. We should be trained in how to relate with different patients and how to adapt our communication to them" (doctor, private setting, cardiology).*

c) *Who is the patient?*

The key barriers to patients being engaged their own healthcare, according to practitioners involved in the study, were mostly related to some patient attitudes and a lack of willingness to get involved. *"Patients should be aware of the diagnosis and what it means ...but if a person is not interested in their own health, nothing can help.' (Nurse, hospital, surgery).*

This is often associated with a general lack of knowledge and awareness amongst patients in relation to their own healthcare and to their own possible involvement in that overall process. This was often described by practitioners in terms of a lack of motivation, lack of interest and passivity denial of illness and lack of commitment to enact a healthy lifestyle. *"The level of education and health literacy is basically one of the most important barrier to effective patient engagement...when the patient is less educated or belong to a disadvantaged socio-cultural environment-...well, in this case it is very difficult to engage him/her..." (nurse, hospital, pneumology).*

Clinicians also considered potential modifiable barriers to patient engagement such as dealing with individuals with poor health literacy or belonging to vulnerable populations; or having some physical impairment. Whilst age and ethnicity are not modifiable factors, the barriers reported by the involved clinicians in relation to the patients' characteristics are linked more to their prejudices that could be managed by sensitizing them or providing educational interventions. For example, some older patients believe that the patients' role should be passive, thus accepting the authority of clinicians, which could be not questioned. *There are some patients – generally the elderly – that prefer to be guided by their doctors. Well, the younger patients are more available to be active in our relationship, but the older ones prefer prescription on what to do or not to do because they think that I am the doctor and I know what they have to do..."* *(doctor, hospital, oncology).* Similarly, unless other reported barriers (i.e. level of education) are relatively non-modifiable, their influence on patient engagement could be mitigated if health professionals provide alternative ways to support patients' change and their active role. Again, also in this case, the strategy for promoting patient engagement could be to act on attitudinal change towards the possibility to act a starring role in the health management.

Regarding the psychological dynamics that occur when patients have to deal with a disease, clinicians underlined that not having time to come to adjust to a diagnosis is a barrier to effective patient engagement. Timing barriers are potentially modifiable barriers for most situations, if we reconsider where active patient engagement might fit in the patients' illness trajectory and if we adopt a processual vision of his/her engagement experience. *"Not all patient should be engaged always. It depends on the moment of their illness...we should identify the best moment to engage them" (nurse, hospital, oncology).*

Strategies to Promote Patient Engagement. HCPs also referred that there are some key areas of interventions particularly recommendable to promote patient engagement in healthcare.

- *Improving patient doctor relationship and shared decision making.* Clinicians strongly highlighted the need to engage patients in a high-quality relationship with them in order to shared care plan which are satisfying for both parts. This kind of partnership approach is recognized by clinicians as a boost for patient engagement. *"Patients, sometimes, need some help to understand the treatment options, and the clinician must communicate risks effectively and elicit and respect patients' preferences and values" (nurse, hospital, cardiology).*
- *Promoting multidisciplinary care approach.* Patient engagement programs that also transform practice organizational culture have been recognized by the involved

clinicians to have greater impact than those requiring the patients to do all the changing. Collaborative multidisciplinary care teams within a practice and care coordination with inpatient, emergency, and specialty services beyond primary care practice walls are particularly important for improving chronic patient engagement in their healthcare journey. *"Taking care of complex patients and assuring their engagement means to strongly support multidisciplinary team that are able to understand them in a holistic way" (nurse, hospital, cardiology).*

- *Using technologies to enhance the patients' active role in the care course.* Interventions adopting some technological components to support the delivery of care, might enhance the engagement experience of chronic patients in the healthcare practitioners' perspective. Health professionals particularly sustained disease self-monitoring tools that encompass the use of devices, audio, video, and other telecommunication technologies to monitor patient status. Health information technologies are considered effective when they "augment" and support, rather then replace, interactions between patients/caregivers and professionals. *"Technologies could be a very relevant tool for empowering and engaging patients in the clinical path...however, to effectively adopt new technologies, the most important thing is the medical staff's awareness of benefits of technological innovation adoption"; "Technologies are relevant but they should not be a alternative of the patient-doctor relationship!" (diabetologist, hospital).*

3.2.3 Being a Health Professional in the Era of Patient Engagement: A Matter of Identity Change

Reflecting upon patient engagement stimulated HCPs to report about changes that this approach to the patient care has implied for their professional identity. HCPs refers that, unless the value of engaging patients is almost clear, this shift of paradigm is hard to be incorporated in routine practice because HCPs are trained and socialized in an approach to care based on the treatment of the symptoms – often in acute settings. This approach is based on the view that the problem is linked to the patient's behavior rather than the HCPs approach to care, which has been seldom considered. Moreover, HCPs referred a substantial gap between the medical training curriculum devoted to promote a highly specialized education and the requirements from the field that implies to adopt a wider and systemic vision of the patient care. Sharing the patient engagement paradigms implies to have wider visions of the patients' care pathway where the presence of multiple professionals is required to reach successful outcomes. *"I had trainings in caring the disease, the organic problem...It is difficult to put into practice a totally different approach where you have to relate with persons and not with organs" (doctor, hospital, surgery).* Adopting a patient engagement view means to *"redefine the power dynamics that occurs in the therapeutic relationship with the patients".* To engage patients means to recognize that in the medical encounters two experts meet each other: one (i.e. the doctor) is the technical expert and the other (i.e. the patient) is the illness experience expert. According to this perspective, the therapeutic relationship should be acknowledged as partnership where patients and clinicians are co-author of the patients' health trajectory. *"In this perspective, we can say that doctors and patients should sit on the same side of the desk looking at the same directions" (doctor, hospital, oncology); "In my opinion, speaking about patient engagement is like being together (patient and clinicians) on the same boat...rowing in the same direction" (nurse, hospital, diabetology).* Moreover, the patient engagement visions need a process of *reframing of the boundaries among disciplines and professions.* Engaging chronic patients in the clinical workflow means to activate collaboration and partnership among all the professionals involved in the patients care, to redistribute duties and promote task shift. *"Engaging patients needs to have a complex vision of his/her clinical course. This means to overcome a fragmented vision of the clinical interventions and to promote multidisciplinary care team, inside and outside the hospital walls" (doctor, hospital, cardiology).*

4 Discussion

This research provides insights into the HCPs' variety of representations linked to patient engagement, their perceived barriers and enablers for its concrete implementation in the clinical practice, and their expectations towards the outcomes of engaging patients. Moreover, the findings also highlighted the effect of the patient engagement paradigm on the health professionals' work identity and the implications for their perceived role.

Firstly, HCPs' representations and meanings related to the concept of patient engagement varied greatly among the involved clinicians. This huge variation is particularly evident when discussing the definition of patient engagement and the contexts in which patient engagement takes place. This finding, on one side confirmed the fragmentation of definitions of patient engagement suggested by other studies that showed how patient engagement is a nuanced concept that include a wide range of patient's activities or behaviors [10–12]. Moreover, this wide spectrum of visions and meanings linked to the concept of patient engagement appears to concern the degree to which patients might (or not) take part in the clinical process. Particularly, it connotes different levels of power transfer from health professionals to patients in the form of increased knowledge and responsibility on health outcomes and illness trajectories. This result confirmed previous studies that highlighted different professional-determined forms of patient participation in their healthcare disposed along a power continuum from information-giving to shared decision making [13–15]. To conceive patient engagement as promoting patient adherence and compliance to treatment underlines a still passivizing logic in the patient-health provider relationship where the doctor took a dominant role and made decisions on behalf of the patient, a 'passive' recipient in the process [16]. Then, when professionals were asked about their perceived benefit of engaging patient in their healthcare they overall refereed a generally positive attitude towards patient engagement because it would lead to improvements in the patients' ability to adequately follow treatments and care prescriptions, along with augmenting the patient's satisfactions and trust towards the relationship with the providers and the healthcare services. This result in aligned with other empirical studies that demonstrated the impact of the patient engagement on a great variety of patients' outcomes [17, 18]. On the other side, results emerged from this study suggested that, although an increasing valorization of patient engagement in healthcare conceived by health professionals as an opportunity to build value both for patients and health organization, this is not necessarily prioritized. This because this practice might fight with other relevant professional values such as responsibility as well as contextual or cultural factors featuring the current medical practice. Moreover, clinicians referred they had little training in how to support patient engagement. This result confirm previous studies that highlighted the lack of medical training devoted to educate clinicians in this area [19, 20]. Clearly, more patient engagement support training for clinicians is needed. Particularly, healthcare professionals recognized new technologies as a promising tool to support greater patient engagement. Yet open questions remain about how they can encourage their adoption and what factors might contribute to sustain their use by patients and caregivers. Furthermore, participants referred a complex system of barriers that might hinder the realization of patient engagement in the medical practice. These barriers are at different levels and mainly refer to: specific patients' characteristics; dynamics occurring in relationship between the patients and the health providers; organizational aspects of the healthcare services. These barriers are coherent with recent frameworks discussed in the literature that suggest to consider elements at different level of complexity to promote patient engagement where technologies are crucial enablers of its implementation [22]. Future work is needed to directly elicit the patients and caregivers' perspectives on strategies to build real patient engagement in healthcare and to test the impact of these strategies on clinical and psychological outcomes.

References

1. Hibbard, J.H., Mahoney, E.: Toward a theory of patient and consumer activation. Patient Educ. Couns. **78**(3), 377–381 (2010)
2. Barello, S., Graffigna, G., Vegni, E.: Patient engagement as an emerging challenge for healthcare services: mapping the literature. Nurs. Res. Pract. 7 (2012)
3. Forbat, L., Cayless, S., Knighting, K., Cornwell, J., Kearney, N.: Engaging patients in health care: an empirical study of the role of engagement on attitudes and action. Patient Educ. Couns. [Internet] **74**(1), 84–90 (2009)
4. Pelletier, L.R., Stichler, J.F.: Action brief: patient engagement and activation: a health reform imperative and improvement opportunity for nursing. Nurs. Outlook [Internet] **61**(1), 51–54 (2013)
5. Hibbard, J.H., Greene, J., Shi, Y., Mittler, J., Scanlon, D.: Taking the long view: how well do patient activation scores predict outcomes four years later? Med. Care Res. Rev. [Internet] **72**, 324 (2015)
6. Alexander, J.A., Hearld, L.R., Mittler, J.N., Harvey, J.: Patient-physician role relationships and patient activation among individuals with chronic illness. Health Serv Res. **47**(3 Pt 1), 1201–1223
7. Graffigna, G., Barello, S., Riva, G.: How to make health information technology effective? The challenge of patient engagement. Arch. Phys. Med. Rehabil. (2013)
8. Graffigna, G., Barello, S., Bonanomi, A., Menichetti, J.: The motivating function of healthcare professional in eHealth and mHealth interventions for type 2 diabetes patients and the mediating role of patient engagement. J. Diabetes Res. **2016** (2016)

9. Barello, S., Graffigna, G., Vegni, E.: Patient engagement as an emerging challenge for healthcare services: mapping the literature. Nurs. Res. Pract. [Internet] **2012**, 1–7 (2012)
10. Gallivan, J., Burns, K.K., Bellows, M., Eigenseher, C.: The many faces of patient engagement. J. Particip. Med. [Internet] **4**, e32 (2012)
11. Sandman, L., Granger, B.B., Ekman, I., Munthe, C.: Adherence, shared decision-making and patient autonomy. Med. Health Care Philos. **15**, 115–127 (2012)
12. Edwards, A., Elwyn, G.: Inside the black box of shared decision making: distinguishing between the process of involvement and who makes the decision. Health Expect [Internet] **9** (4), 307–320 (2006). http://www.ncbi.nlm.nih.gov/pubmed/17083558
13. Barello, S., Graffigna, G.: Engagement-sensitive decision making: training doctors to sustain patient engagement in medical consultations. Patient Engagement: Consum.-Centered Model Innovate Healthcare (2016)
14. Kaba, R., Sooriakumaran, P.: The evolution of the doctor-patient relationship. Int. J. Surg. **5**, 57–65 (2007)
15. Remmers, C., Hibbard, J., Mosen, D.M., Wagenfield, M., Hoye, R.E., Jones, C.: Is patient activation associated with future health outcomes and healthcare utilization among patients with diabetes? J. Ambul Care Manag. **32**(4), 320–327 (2009)
16. Hibbard, J.H., Mahoney, E.R., Stock, R., Tusler, M.: Do increases in patient activation result in improved self-management behaviors? Health Serv. Res. **42**(4), 1443–1463 (2007)
17. Graffigna, G., Barello, S., Bonanomi, A.: The role of patient health engagement model (PHE-model) in affecting patient activation and medication adherence: a structural equation model. PLoS One **12**(6) (2017)
18. Barello, S., Graffigna, G., Pitacco, G., et al.: An educational intervention to train professional nurses in promoting patient engagement: a pilot feasibility study. Front. Psychol. 2020 (2017)
19. Greene, J., Sacks, R.M., Hibbard, J.H., Overton, V.: How much do clinicians support patient self-management? The development of a measure to assess clinician self-management support. Healthcare [Internet] (2016)
20. Graffigna, G., Barello, S., Riva, G., Savarese, M., Menichetti, J., Castelnuovo, G., et al.: Fertilizing a patient engagement ecosystem to innovate healthcare: toward the first Italian consensus conference on patient engagement. Front. Psychol. **8**(Jun), 1–6 (2017)

Investigating Prosodic Accommodation in Clinical Interviews with Depressed Patients

Brian Vaughan[1(✉)], Carolina De Pasquale[1], Lorna Wilson[2], Charlie Cullen[3], and Brian Lawlor[4]

[1] Dublin Institute of Technology, Dublin, Ireland
brian.vaughan@dit.ie
[2] St. James's University Hospital Dublin, Dublin, Ireland
[3] University of the West of Scotland, Hamilton, Scotland
[4] Trinity College Dublin, Dublin, Ireland

Abstract. Six in-depth clinical interviews, involving six elderly female patients (aged 60+) and one female psychiatrist, were recorded and analysed for a number of prosodic accommodation variables. Our analysis focused on pitch, speaking time, and vowel-space ratio. Findings indicate that there is a dynamic manifestation of prosodic accommodation over the course of the interactions. There is clear adaptation on the part of the psychiatrist, even going so far as to have a reduced vowel-space ratio, mirroring a reduced vowel-space ratio in the depressed patients. Previous research has found a reduced vowel-space ratio to be associated with psychological distress; however, we suggest that it indicates a high level of adaptation on the part of the psychiatrist and needs to be considered when analysing psychiatric clinical interactions.

Keywords: Speech analysis · Clinical interviews · Depression
Prosody · Accommodation · Interaction · Vowel-space

1 Introduction

Clinical depression is a common illness with a negative impact on several aspects of a patient's life, accounting for 4.3% of the global burden of disease, and is among the single largest contributor to global disability [1]. In Europe, depression has a 9% prevalence among men and a 17% prevalence among women; the economic costs of depression amounts to 136.3 billion Euro in the European Economic Area [2]. There are some objectively measurable markers for depression [3], but none that can be unobtrusively and readily measured during diagnosis, which at this time depends on subjective assessments by expert practitioners. These practitioners have to rely on patients' self-reported symptoms and have to perform clinical interviews to assess the impact and prevalence of symptoms on the individual [4]. In an effort to find an easily measured objective marker for depression, recent studies have explored the impact that it has on a number

© ICST Institute for Computer Sciences, Social Informatics and Telecommunications Engineering 2018
P. Cipresso et al. (Eds.): MindCare 2018, LNICST 253, pp. 150–159, 2018.
https://doi.org/10.1007/978-3-030-01093-5_19

of prosodic variables, which are affected by a variety of symptoms that occur in depressed individuals, such as psychomotor retardation, muscle tension and cognitive impairment [5]; indeed, changes to the prosodic behaviour of individuals with mental health issues are well known (for a review see [5]). These studies have found that depression induces measurable, manifest changes in a person's speech that can be indicative of depressive severity or even suicidal ideation. Some of the symptoms required for a diagnosis of depression can lead to a variety of behaviours that impact interactions. Individuals affected by a loss of motivation can experience social withdrawal, excessive negative thoughts, and feelings of guilt, which can lead to socio-communicative disruptive behaviours. During an interaction, participants will subconsciously adapt their communicative behaviour to that of their interlocutor, a phenomenon that is described using many terms, particularly prosodic adaptation, accommodation, synchrony, mimicry, convergence, alignment and entrainment [6]. Prosodic accommodation occurs between speakers when changes in their prosodic parameters move in synchronous alignment or when they converge towards a common point [7], and is an important factor in social interactions, as it aids comprehension and understanding between participants [8].

2 Speech and Depression

Various researchers have found that depression results in measurable changes in prosody (tone, intensity and rhythm of the voice); these changes have been found to be somewhat indicative of the severity of depression and have been used to differentiate between depressed and non-depressed patients. Moore et al. found that pitch, energy and speech rate feature statistics could be used to differentiate between patients with depression from those without [9]. Likewise, Cannizzaro et al. found speaking rate and pitch variability to be strongly negatively correlated with the severity of major depression [10]. Ozdas et al. observed that jitter (short-term perturbations of pitch) are different in patients at imminent risk of suicide[1] as compared to those in a control group of non-depressed patients. Moreover, they developed a Machine Learning (ML) classifier, using these findings, which performed well in discriminating between suicidal speech and speech from the control group [11]. Similarly, France et al. were able to discriminate between the speech of depressed patients and the speech of suicidal patients using prosodic analysis [12].

While interpersonal effects have not been investigated to the same extent, promising results have been obtained in some studies. Yang et al. observed that, as the severity of a patients depression changed, so too did the prosodic parameters of the trained clinical interviewers interviewing the patient. They suggest that the observed effect is not simply caused by behavioural mimicry, but rather a reflection of how the "pitch", measured by the fundamental frequency (f_0), is influenced by the intentions and goals of the speaker (in this case, to express

---

[1] These patients comprised of people who had recorded suicide notes and people who had subsequently made potentially lethal suicide attempts.

sympathy). Scherer et al. found that vowel-space was reduced in depression, post-traumatic stress disorder (PTSD), and suicidality. Vowel-space is defined as the frequency space covered by the first and second formants of the vowels /i/, /a/, and /u/ as these are at the extremes of a triangular shaped frequency space [13]. Scherer et al. [14] also found that the interviewers' acoustic features were strongly correlated with the depression severity of the interaction partner: interviewers' f_0 mean and variability were correlated to the partner's depression severity, and interviewers displayed a "breathy" voice quality (associated with a more empathetic demeanour, and with sad behaviours [14]). The findings of both Yang and Scherer, as discussed above, suggest that an interviewer's behaviour might also be an indicator of the depression severity of the interviewee, and thus merits further investigation.

2.1 Prosodic Accommodation

While the majority of research on prosodic accommodation describes it as a mono-tonic communicative property, recent work has demonstrated that prosodic accommodation is a dynamic phenomenon that increases and decreases over the course of an interaction [8,15]. Moreover, the dynamic manifestation of prosodic accommodation is directly related to the perceived naturalness of conversational flow, mutual understanding and affinity, and the overall level of engagement between speakers. Studies on the effects of depression on speech and prosodic characteristics tend to focus on the individual speech parameters of the depressed patient and their interlocutor, and neglect the socio-communicative aspect of prosodic accommodation. Previous work has shown this to be a dynamic, socio-communicative process that is indicative of the level of engagement and communication between interlocutors, and demonstrated that higher levels of prosodic accommodation were associated with a higher level of engagement and greater affinity between interlocutors [8]. Prosodic accommodation was found to be positively correlated with the level of communication and global coordination between interlocutors. Previous research also found that interlocutors accommodate across a range of prosodic parameters: intensity [16], speech rate [17,18], and pitch [19]. Collins [20] and Gregory et al. [21] observed global pitch to be indicative of a level of accommodation (in terms of mean f_0), using unconstrained conversations and interviews of English. Accommodation in average vocal intensity and intensity range has been observed both at the global and local levels of task-based and unconstrained dialogues of English and Swedish [15,22]. Accommodation is important in decreasing communicative misunderstandings, and facilitating faster goal attainment [23–25], while also increasing the level of rapport and overall social success of an interaction [26–28].

3   Methodology

In order to investigate prosodic accommodation in psychiatrist/patient interactions, noise-free, channel separated audio recordings were needed. Six psychiatrist/patient interviews were recorded over the course of a few weeks, at an outpatient clinic for elderly sufferers of depression at St. James's Hospital Dublin; patients were six elderly female individuals (aged 60+). Ethics approval was sought and granted from the hospital. All participant data was anonymised: participants were assigned coded names (participant 1, 2, 3 etc), and all medical records, including details on the depressive disorders, remained with the psychiatrist and hospital. Only basic demographic data was collected alongside the speech recordings (duration of the disorder, number of major episodes, age, and gender). All participants were broadly classed by the psychiatrists as mild to severely depressed, with no comorbid cognitive impairment (scores >24 on the Mini-Mental State Examination); HAM-D scores were not obtained, this is an aspect that future work will address, by ensuring a more granular measure of depression is captured and used as part of the analysis. The average length of the recordings was 20 min. In order to preserve the normal psychiatrist/patient interview environment, it was important to ensure that any recording set-up was as non-intrusive as possible. To this end, a small, portable audio recorder, the ZOOM H4N, was used, in conjunction with discrete clip-on lapel mics. No constraints were placed on the topics of conversation; the clinical interviews were part of the normal course of treatment for all participants and were not in addition to ongoing treatment.

Due to the nature of the recordings in the clinical setting, a lot of cross talk was present between channels: the setting and the physical space in which the recording took place did not allow for the speakers to be sufficiently acoustically isolated from each other; therefore, each microphone captured both speakers, albeit at different amplitudes. This made it necessary to prepare the audio for analysis before feature extraction, so that each speaker was clearly labelled and could be separated into different audio channels, and overlapping speech and extraneous noise removed. Each recording was annotated using Textgrids in PRAAT, and where then exported as separated audio files. This ensured that we had noise-free, channel separated audio, ready to be analysed.

4 Analysis

Once the files were separated, acoustic features and prosodic accommodation measures were extracted and computed using Vocavio Matlab software [29][2], and the COVAREP Matlab toolbox [30]. This is a set of open source Matlab scripts for extracting and computing a number of acoustic features. f_0 (pitch) was the main focus of our analysis; as per [7,8], it has long been observed that conversation partners exhibit similar pitch and intonation contours, and f_0 contours are the basis of the AUC calculations (discussed below); moreover, other frequency based components, f_1 and f_2 measurements, are the basis of the vowel-space calculations, which are also discussed below. Intensity based measures and their relation to frequency based measures are currently being explored.

---

[2] http://vocavio.com/.

A Time Aligned Moving Average (TAMA) method [31] was used to obtain a smoother prosodic contour for analysis. In the TAMA method, moving overlapping windows, large enough to extract useful chunks of speech, are used to extract prosodic parameters. Average values for a number of prosodic parameters are calculated for each window, then the window is moved so that the new time window overlaps by a certain degree with the old window (see Fig. 1): the result is a smoother contour, with no significant loss of accuracy in the capture of prosodic dynamics. For our analysis, we used a window length of ten seconds, with a five second overlap. The TAMA method solves the problem of measuring accommodation in conversations, as speakers do not accommodate immediately due the reactive temporal nature of conversation, and their inherent turn-based structure.

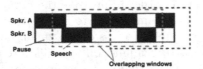

Fig. 1. Time Aligned Moving Window. The diagram illustrates the TAMA method, showing how the moving windows operate.

From each average obtained with the TAMA method, a correlation window of thirty seconds was used to calculate the correlation of prosodic measures in the dyad. The level of accommodation in dyads are measured with the Spearman's correlation coefficient $\rho\epsilon[-1,1]$. Large $\rho_{xy} \gg 0$ can be considered indicators of high levels of accommodation, while small $\rho_{xy} \ll 0$ indicate a low level of accommodation [32]. Our TAMA settings, of a window length of ten seconds, with a five second overlap, resulted in six values per 30 second correlation window. As per [32] a normalised area-under-curve (AUC) calculation is used to make an approximate comparison between the two speakers regarding the similarity of their pitch contours over the course of an interaction; this is taken to be an indication of the balance of effort of each speaker in adapting their prosodic parameters such that a larger AUC indicates stronger changes in pitch by the speaker. The normalised values were obtained by dividing the individual AUC calculations with the summed AUC of both speakers, and then multiplied by 100; this gives individual percentage values, enabling differences to be expressed as a percentage of overall effort:

$$\text{NORM}_{auc}^{A} = \frac{auc^{A}}{auc^{A} + auc^{B}} * 100 \tag{1}$$

where aucA is the AUC for speaker A and aucB is the AUC for speaker B. The combined $\text{NORM}_{auc}^{A} + \text{NORM}_{auc}^{B}$ will always be equal to 100 percent. Formant analysis and vowel-space calculations were carried out using the COVAREP Matlab toolbox [30], as per [13]. Speaking time was calculated for each speaker using an intensity based Voice Activity Detector (VAD), with the intensity threshold set to a level that ensured all speech was accurately extracted. The overall speaking time for each speaker was calculated as a percentage of total speaking time for each conversation.

5 Results

5.1 Pitch

All the conversations are positively correlated. There are no particularly strong values (close to +1), and the overall accommodation level across all conversations is weak (see Table 1 for overall accommodation values). More pertinent, however, is the fact that the dynamic nature of prosodic accommodation means that there will be moments of high and low accommodation throughout, so a single accommodation score will not capture this dynamic aspect, as discussed in Sect. 2.1). This dynamic aspect is evident from the graphical representations of the accommodation of each interaction, which show a huge variation in pitch accommodation level. Section 2.1 shows a graphical representation from one conversation that is typical of all the conversations: moments of high and low pitch accommodation throughout and an overall high degree of variability (Fig. 2).

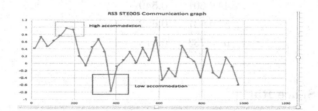

Fig. 2. Accommodation Graph. The graph shows the accommodation dynamics of the dyad: clear moments of high and low accommodation can be observed (highlighted), showing that accommodation during the clinical interactions was dynamic.

5.2 AUC and Speaking Time

The area-under-the-curve (AUC) calculations (see Sect. 4), show that in two of the six conversations, the psychiatrist made most of the effort to adapt to the patient. In two of the six conversations, the patient was making the most effort to accommodate. In two conversations, there is a fairly even balance of effort between the psychiatrist and patient. In all conversations the patient was doing the majority of the talking. Table 1 shows the overall accommodation scores and the speaking time and AUC value for each of the six conversations. The reduced speaking time across all interactions of the psychiatrist can potentially be explained by the nature of the clinical interaction, where the psychiatrist asks questions that are then answered at length by the patient (Table 2).

Table 1. Table showing the overall accommodation for each interaction, as well as speaking time, and AUC values for the patient and psychiatrist in each interaction.

	Team accom.	Speaking time			AUC Values	
		Overall	Patient	Psychiatrist	Patient	Psychiatrist
1	0.106259	67%	49%	18%	35%	65%
2	0.199743	66%	42%	25%	70%	30%
3	0.184069	70%	53%	16%	47%	53%
4	0.305988	71%	56%	15%	52%	48%
5	0.108911	61%	35%	26%	44%	56%
6	0.0716094	69%	53%	16%	58%	42%

Table 2. Table of the vowel-space ratios for patients and psychiatrist. No vowel-space reduction would be a 1:1 ratio. Values less that this indicate a reduction in vowel-space.

	Vowel space ratio values	
	Patient	Psychiatrist
1	0.607	0.612
2	0.496	0.673
3	0.451	0.409
4	0.601	0.549
5	0.637	0.662
6	0.733	0.618

5.3   Vowel Space Ratio

In agreement with [13], observed vowel space ratio was reduced in the patients' speech: this preliminary result supports their findings of reduced vowel-space in depressed patients. However, analysis also showed significant reduction in the vowel space ratio of the psychiatrist involved in the interactions. While Scherer et al. did find some vowel space ratio reduction in non-depressed participants [13], what is potentially significant about our results is the consistency across all interactions. Vowel-space ratio reduction on the part of the psychiatrist has not been previously investigated, and it represents a potential indication of adaptive behaviour in response to that of the patient. Due to ethical requirements, it is extremely unlikely that a depressed psychiatrist would practice and care for depressed patients, therefore it is more likely that the vowel-space reduction in the psychiatrist's speech indicates a global measure of prosodic accommodation.

6   Discussion and Future Work

Our investigation shows that prosodic accommodation occurs in clinical interactions, and is a dynamic phenomenon, as per previous findings (see Sect. 2.1).

Using a combination of speaking time and normalised AUC values, we show that, in two of the six conversations, the psychiatrist is making the most effort to accommodate; in two of the conversations the patient makes the most effort, and in two conversations there is a balance of effort. There is no clear reason for the variance in effort across conversations; it is possible that a more granular measure of depression could account for these variances, with increased depression severity being linked to a reduced AUC value. This is an aspect of the results that will be further investigated.

Vowel-space ratio measurements are more consistent, and the results suggest that vowel-space ratio may be used as a measure of global interpersonal adaptation in the context of clinical interaction; vowel-space ratio has not been investigated as a measure of prosodic adaptation, and this result will be explored further. We must also consider possible age related effects across all parameters, but especially vowel space ratio measures, as there may be age related aspects that can cause a reduced vowel-space ratio. However, given the age difference between the patients and the psychiatrist (25+years), age related effects were not likely a factor in her reduced vowel space ratio, even if they were for the patient group. Moreover, even if patient vowel-space ratio was reduced due to age related effects, the reduced vowel-space ratio of the psychiatrist can still be indicative of strong adaptation on her part. Further work will be conducted with a more granular measurement of depression severity (using the Hamilton depression rating scale (HAM-D) [33]), as well as an age and gender matched control group. Future work will also focus on further examining vowel-space ratio reduction across a larger data-set of psychiatrist/patient interactions, as well as exploring the relationship between speaking time and AUC calculations, and their relation to aspects of the conversation, such as topic, and depression severity.

References

1. World Health Organization: Depression and other common mental disorders: global health estimates. Technical report, World Health Organization, Geneva (2017)
2. Smit, F., Shields, L., Petrea, I.: Preventing depression in the WHO European region. Technical report, World Health Organization (2016)
3. Strawbridge, R., Young, A.H., Cleare, A.J.: Biomarkers for depression: recent insights, current challenges and future prospects. Neuropsychiatr. Dis. Treat. **13**, 1245–1262 (2017)
4. Asgari, M., Shafran, I., Sheeber, L.B.: Inferring clinical depression from speech and spoken utterances. In: 2014 IEEE International Workshop on Machine Learning for Signal Processing (MLSP), pp. 1–5. IEEE, September 2014
5. Cummins, N., Scherer, S., Krajewski, J., Schnieder, S., Epps, J., Quatieri, T.F.: A review of depression and suicide risk assessment using speech analysis. Speech Commun. **71**, 10–49 (2015)
6. De Looze, C., Oertel, C., Rauzy, S., Campbell, N.: Measuring dynamics of mimicry. In: ICPhS, vol. 1, pp. 1294–1297, August 2011

7. De Looze, C., Rauzy, S.: Measuring speakers' similarity in speech by means of prosodic cues: methods and potential. In: Proceedings of the Annual Conference of the International Speech Communication Association, INTERSPEECH, pp. 1393–1396 (2011)
8. De Looze, C., Scherer, S., Vaughan, B., Campbell, N.: Investigating automatic measurements of prosodic accommodation and its dynamics in social interaction. Speech Commun. **58**, 11–34 (2014)
9. Moore II, E., Clements, M., Peifer, J., Weisser, L.: Analysis of prosodic variation in speech for clinical depression. In: Proceedings of the 25th Annual International Conference of the IEEE Engineering in Medicine and Biology Society (IEEE Cat. No. 03CH37439), vol. 3, pp. 2925–2928 (2003)
10. Cannizzaro, M.S., Harel, B., Reilly, N., Chappell, P., Snyder, P.J.: Voice acoustical measurement of the severity of major depression. Brain Cogn. **56**, 30–35 (2004)
11. Ozdas, A., Shiavi, R., Silverman, S., Silverman, M., Wilkes, D.: Analysis of fundamental frequency for near term suicidal risk assessment. In: SMC 2000 Conference Proceedings. 2000 IEEE International Conference on Systems, Man and Cybernetics. 'Cybernetics Evolving to Systems, Humans, Organizations, and Their Complex Interactions' (Cat. No. 00CH37166), vol. 3, pp. 1853–1858. IEEE (2000)
12. France, D.J., Shiavi, R.G., Silverman, S., Silverman, M., Wilkes, D.M.: Acoustical properties of speech as indicators of depression and suicidal risk. IEEE Trans. Biomed. Eng. **47**, 829–837 (2000)
13. Scherer, S., Morency, L.-P., Gratch, J., Pestian, J.: Reduced vowel space is a robust indicator of psychological distress: a cross-corpus analysis. In: 2015 IEEE International Conference on Acoustics, Speech and Signal Processing (ICASSP), pp. 4789–4793. IEEE, April 2015
14. Scherer, S., Hammal, Z., Yang, Y., Morency, L.-P., Cohn, J.F.: Dyadic behavior analysis in depression severity assessment interviews. In: Proceedings of the 16th International Conference on Multimodal Interaction - ICMI 2014, pp. 112–119 (2014)
15. Levitan, R., Hirschberg, J.: Measuring acoustic-prosodic entrainment with respect to multiple levels and dimensions. In: Proceedings of Interspeech 2011, pp. 3081–3084. ISCA (2011)
16. Coulston, R., Oviatt, S., Darves, C.: Amplitude convergence in children's conversational speech with animated personas. In: 7th International Conference on Spoken Language Processing, ICSLP 2002 - INTERSPEECH 2002 (2002)
17. Kousidis, S., Dorran, D., McDonnell, C., Coyle, E.: Times series analysis of acoustic feature convergence in human dialogues. In: Proceedings of Interspeech (2008)
18. Edlund, J., Heldner, M., Hirschberg, J.: Pause and gap length in face-to-face interaction. In: Proceedings of the Annual Conference of the International Speech Communication Association, INTERSPEECH, pp. 2779–2782 (2009)
19. Babel, M., Bulatov, D.: The role of fundamental frequency in phonetic accommodation. Lang. Speech **55**, 231–248 (2011)
20. Collins, B.: Convergence of fundamental frequencies in conversation: if it happens, does it matter? In: Proceedings of ICSLP, vol. 98, (1998)
21. Gregory, S.W., Webster, S.: A nonverbal signal in voices of interview partners effectively predicts communication accommodation and social status perceptions. J. Pers. Soc. Psychol. **70**(6), 1231–1240 (1996)
22. Heldner, M., Edlund, J.: Pauses, gaps and overlaps in conversations. J. Phon. **38**, 555–568 (2010)
23. Parrill, F., Kimbara, I.: Seeing and hearing double: the influence of mimicry in speech and gesture on observers. J. Nonverbal Behav. **30**, 157–166 (2006)

24. Pickering, M.J., Garrod, S.: Alignment as the basis for successful communication. Res. Lang. Comput. **4**, 203–228 (2006)
25. Boylan, P.: Accommodation Theory Revisited Again. Lingua e società, pp. 287–305 (2009)
26. Tickle-Degnen, L., Rosenthal, R.: The nature of rapport and its nonverbal correlates. Psychol. Inq. **1**(4), 285–293 (1990)
27. Shepard, C., Giles, H., Le Poire, B.: Communication accommodation theory. In: Robinson, W., Giles, H. (eds.) The New Handbook of Language and Social Psychology, pp. 33–56. Wiley, New York (2001)
28. Miles, L.K., Nind, L.K., Macrae, C.N.: The rhythm of rapport: interpersonal synchrony and social perception. J. Exp. Soc. Psychol. **45**(3), 585–589 (2009)
29. Vocavio (2017)
30. Degottex, G., Kane, J., Drugman, T., Raitio, T., Scherer, S.: COVAREP - a collaborative voice analysis repository for speech technologies. In: 2014 IEEE International Conference on Acoustics, Speech and Signal Processing (ICASSP), pp. 960–964. IEEE, May 2014
31. Kousidis, S., Dorran, D., McDonell, C., Coyle, E.: Time series analysis of acoustic feature convergence in human dialogues. In: Specom 2009, St. Petersburg, Russian Federation, pp. 1–6 (2009)
32. De Looze, C., Vaughan, B., Kelly, F., Kay, A.: Providing objective metrics of team communication skills via interpersonal coordination mechanisms. In: INTERSPEECH, Dresden, Germany, pp. 1–5 (2015)
33. Hamilton, M.: Development of a rating scale for primary depressive illness. Br. J. Soc. Clin. Psychol. **6**, 278–96 (1967)

Author Index

Printed in the United States
By Bookmasters